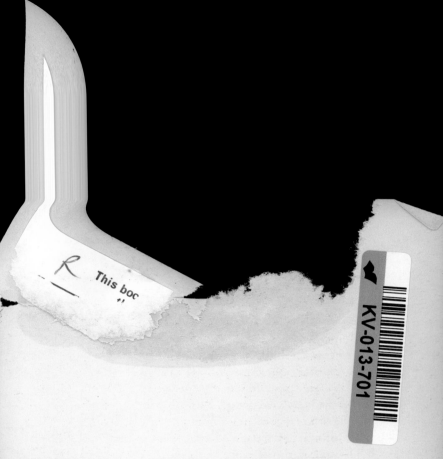

Belinda Grant N.D., D.O., Dip. C., has a commitment to natural healthcare and personal growth which began in her early twenties when she first consulted a naturopath. Since then she has studied and worked with many forms of healing, incorporating them into her natural health practice. She is the author of the best-selling *Detox Diet Book* and lives and works in London where she also teaches and makes occasional radio broadcasts.

A–Z of Natural Healthcare

BELINDA GRANT

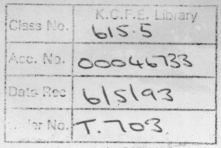
An OPTIMA book

First published in Great Britain in 1993 by Optima

A CIP catalogue record for this book
is available from the British Library

ISBN 0 356 20982 2

Typeset by Leaper & Gard Ltd, Bristol, England
Printed in England by Clays Ltd, St Ives plc

Optima Books
A Division of
Little, Brown and Company (UK) Limited
165 Great Dover Street
London SE1 4YA

DEDICATION

To Mr and Mrs Reinstein,
my great and generous friends.

CONTENTS

ACKNOWLEDGEMENTS

Betty Balcombe has been an inspiration throughout the writing of this book and the chapter on healing was written as a result of interviews with her. Many friends and colleagues also gave generously of their time with advice and comments on their own specialist subjects, and I would particularly like to thank Neil Pilkington.

Nora, my mother, gave her love, support and encouragement throughout and Sandra Boyes demystified the computer process for me and was there whenever I needed help.

INTRODUCTION

This book is about one wide-ranging, comprehensive system of healthcare. It is not interventionist, not invasive, but supportive, life-enhancing and, often, simple.

The therapies are listed in alphabetical order and contain information on natural forms of healthcare, methods of treatment and practices. The aim is to provide a reference for self-help and information; many chapters include practical help and advice for managing and treating minor ailments. The therapy sections also outline what each particular area of speciality has to offer, and what you can expect from a visit to a practitioner.

Alternative medicine is such a huge umbrella, containing many different ways of approaching individual health and a variety of practical applications. This book contains information on all those therapies which support the body's natural function – its self-regulating mechanisms; and most of these have home applications.

I believe it is as important for people to be able to make informed choices about their healthcare as in every other area of life, and with the rich abundance of therapies currently available, our need for information is greater than ever. Even those who have consulted a practitioner may want to know more about how and why their treatments work. In order for any healing to occur, an understanding of the nature of the problem is imperative. In the true spirit of holism, recognising the strength of the body–mind connection, any physical action without conscious appreciation of its purpose can only be partly effective.

This A–Z attempts to offer a comprehensive guide to the many natural options available to us. Under their own umbrella of naturopathy, a wide variety of approaches and skills are to be found. Not least among the reasons for such choice is one of the primary objectives of this philosophy – that the work is not so much in curing the patient, as in educating them to live in harmony with their own unique recipe for health.

NATURAL
HEALTHCARE

Natural healthcare provides a myriad of different ways of restoring balance to all levels of our being. Its three main 'arms' or areas of concern are with the person's physical structure (see Manipulative therapies, Kinesiology, Bodywork, Massage, etc.); how their body works (see Dietary care, Herbs, Juicing, etc.); and the links between the psycho-emotional and the physical (see Body forms, Counselling, Energywork, Healing, etc.).

Many of these healing techniques have been known to us for centuries. Eating herbs with a meal for their medicinal properties stemmed from learning the therapeutic values of all locally grown foods. From the time our ancestors were hunter-gatherers, we have known the importance of remaining physically active and of moderating and varying our food intake. And, as social animals, we have always known the value of sharing our thoughts, ideas and feelings with others.

Some of the therapies and practices included here have evolved more recently. Neuro-linguistic programming (NLP) (see Leading Edge Therapies) and cranio-sacral therapy, (see Cranial Therapy) for example, embrace very new age concepts of holism and effectiveness, yet their roots are firmly planted in the history of healing. As practitioners and patients bring their own individual skills together, and as we continue to push back the limits of our understanding about the magnificence and variety of human experience, so new therapies are born.

In recent years, we in the West have adopted a particular form of medicine and made it mainstream. Allopathic medicine is now accepted as the norm in terms of healthcare – it is what the GP or the MD whom we visit practices, and it is what all our hospitals provide. We have come to know it as medicine, yet it is only one branch of our vast tree of knowledge concerning health.

With an ever-growing awareness of ourselves as multi-dimensional beings with emotional, spiritual, physical and social needs, we realise how these distinct areas of our lives all overlap and influence each other. All the therapies in this book share a view of the individual as comprising more than just a physical body, and the belief that the integrity of *all* parts of a person is central to their health.

Witness the sick person who, in our hospital system, must move from one department to another; from one specialist to another; even from one bed to another in a different ward to have parts of themselves fixed. This is not an argument against specialisation *per se*, more a regret that the cost in this situation seems to be perspective, and patient care. That the whole of humanity is infinitely greater than the sum of its parts seems to have been forgotten in the allopathic system. (Or possibly even proved to be unscientific!) This missing element is what characterises the holistic approach.

The idea that full health involves psycho-emotional and spiritual, as well as physical, well-being is by no means new. Hippocrates spoke at length about the integrity of the individual and the importance of assessing and understanding the person as a whole being, rather than concentrating on the nature of any disease. In taking the Hippocratic oath, allopathic medics have taken only part of a truth and used it out of context; taken an active principle and disregarded the rest.

Of course, not all natural therapies offer a comprehensive approach, but with few exceptions they recognise the existence and importance of an overview. Simple, life-supporting techniques have few side effects, and most are complementary in both senses – they not only enhance the health of the individual, but can work effectively alongside one another. Combining the use of aromatherapy oils with flower remedies and herbs, for example, would be safe, effective and pleasant.

All naturopathic therapies seek to strengthen and support the individual's own life-force or vitality. Through harnessing natural elements and developing ways of working with them, we uncover a system of medicine that is safe, complete, effective and accessible – we can all use it everyday if we need to. The use of diet, herbs, water, physical contact, etc., forms a natural method of primary healthcare, providing everyday solutions to everyday difficulties.

Naturopathy also looks to the maintenance of full health and, as such, forms an important prevention against disease by searching out the underlying causes of any imbalance rather than focusing on any presenting symptoms. We cannot be healthy in isolation; the effects of the environment – pollutants, and food additives such as preservatives, colourings, flavourings, emulsifiers, bleaches and stabilisers – all influence the way in which we function.

The continual need to fight airborne pollutants and other allergens can lead to our immune system being over-taxed. The presence in the diet of adulterated and refined foods can soon lead to poor digestion and assimilation of nutrients, and great internal confusion at a biochemical level. Such physiological stress can lead in turn to faulty elimination and a lack of tone and vitality in the tissues and cells.

It is at this stage that we may begin to manifest 'sub-clinical' feelings of tiredness – feeling below par, a general malaise without any specific complaint. Such under-functioning tissues are also fertile soil for viruses and bacteria.

We are not, as a rule, given enough information about the things that we consume. Nor are we generally educated as to how our bodies work. Although we all have individual differences, the majority of our 'workings' are the same, and a fundamental aspect of natural healthcare is its teaching role. It is easier to make decisions as to our immediate environment, our diet, even our social habits if we understand when and in what form we need them. How many of us would choose, for instance, to deprive ourselves of sunshine? Yet we often attribute a low priority in our schedules to time spent outdoors. And where on the school curriculum are the personal development skills of self-awareness and analysis?

It is often left to the individual, in their search for personal growth, to discover a spiritual aspect to their lives; to understand their own psychology and, particularly in our society, to learn the value and importance of self-nourishment.

Whatever we call our basic vitality – Chi (China), Ki (Japan), Prana (India) or spirit – it is the spark, the energy of life. As living, evolving organisms we are always looking towards full health and the more ways we can find to enhance and facilitate this move, the better. In our quest for optimum health, ease of function and well-being, it is not intervention, but support that is needed.

In listening to our individual needs on all levels, we can begin to find ways to encourage our momentum towards full health. When a symptom of ill health manifests, we can choose to ignore it or see it as a sign pointing the way towards an area in need of our attention. We can liken the body (our physical home) to a house (our material home). On discovering a crack in one of the walls of our house, we would have a number of options – to cover it over with a coat of paint, for example; or to investigate and see whether there might be some subsidence, or shaky foundations.

The choice may well be governed by our sense of responsibility. In our own home, such a crack may lead us to pursue many avenues to ascertain whether there were, indeed, any structural problems; or if it was a simple case of bad decorating skills. Alternatively, we might just phone the landlords and let them know about it.

This analogy reflects so well the attitude that many of us have towards our own health – we can embody our lives, or see them as someone else's responsibility.

A mainstay of the nature-cure philosophy is that health is an individual process and an individual responsibility. The life-force is neither conscious will that may be determined, nor is it unconscious thought and available to our understanding. Yet it exists, and to intervene in its process is a big responsibility. Such intervention requires careful management and may even raise a moral question.

Surgery can be seen as the ultimate in interventionist treatment – vital and life-saving on occasion, an invasive assault nevertheless. Medication is somewhat more insidious because many pharmaceutical drugs interfere with the body's own natural and useful pathways. Pain killers, for example, do nothing to relieve the condition, they just block our awareness of the pain. This has always seemed a little bit like hearing a baby cry and going out to buy a pair of ear plugs. Or moving into a home with an elegant alarm system and working hard to disconnect it as soon as one of the bells goes off.

Intervention, then, may be seen as a serious move – warranted on occasion, but needing to be treated with respect and placed in its proper perspective. It is not the answer if there is an easier, simpler way. Some alternative therapies can also be seen as invasive or interventionist – those that routinely puncture or burn the skin; or that override the person's conscious process. This book adheres to the holistic philosophy of nature cure and explores only those therapies that do not violate the integrity of the individual.

There are, of course, many other systems of healthcare: Kahuna healing; Ayurvedic medicine; Shamanism, homeopathy, to name but a few – naturopathy does not have all the answers for everybody, but it can do a lot! In its simplicity it is deeply impressive; not just in its efficacy, but also in the ease by which it can be used by so many people.

HOW TO USE THIS BOOK

Each alphabetical entry defines a particular natural therapy or practice. In some instances more than one therapy is covered, for example chiropractic, McTimoney technique and osteopathy are all included as Manipulative Therapies; both Alexander technique and the Feldenkrais method are described within Postural Therapies. In some instances, the information from one chapter overlaps with others: Herbs, for example, have their own entry, and are also included as a useful aid to Hydrotherapy and their oils are discussed separately as Aromatherapy.

Whether the therapies involve visits to a practitioner or are designed for more individual use, many of the chapters include suggestions and techniques that can be practised on one's own, without recourse to an expert. In the main these are first-aid tips and reference tables to assist with minor complaints. Obviously, these cannot replace the individually tailored advice available through consultation with a naturopath or other healthcare practitioner.

Many of the suggestions in this book are not, however, about any specific therapy, but are a part of living life in good health. Our need for quiet, outdoor contact and the company of others, for example, can often be as essential to our own well-being as more defined health measures.

Where possible, each chapter suggests books on the subject, and where to find out more. Through the sterling work of the Airlift Book Company and other similar organisations, many American books can now be found in our shops. I have therefore been able to include a wide range of titles and some definitive works. The colleges and professional bodies should all be able to provide a list of practitioners who have completed their courses, details of their curricula and information leaflets.

Finding a practitioner must always be a matter of personal concern – most professional associations will hold a register of those who have graduated from their course, but although professional training is obviously important, it is not the only factor that should govern your choice. Not all practitioners join their relevant associations on qualifying, sometimes for political reasons, sometimes for practical reasons; or experienced practitioners may let their membership lapse. Any areas of expertise or speciality, experience and the rapport you establish with the therapist are all important. By far the best way to find a practitioner is through person referral, but if this is not possible, then use any association's lists as a starting point and interview the practitioner in an initial phone call or short appointment.

Your health and your body are among your greatest assets. It is worth taking time to find the right person who will be sympathetic to your needs and be able to provide you with professional care and advice.

PART ONE

The Therapies

AFFIRMATIONS

These techniques for encouraging change and affirming or enlivening a vision may be verbal, mental or written.

Affirmations can take many forms. Simply, they are an aid to establishing new ways of being, or focusing the individual on a specific thing. 'Every day in every way I'm getting better' is a classic example, albeit a rather global one. Affirmations or 'Positive Thought Repetitions' (PTRs) are often most effective when extremely specific, and it helps if they are time-related too, e.g. 'Today's the day ...' or 'Now is the time for ...'.

These sayings can be thought aloud, written out or focused on silently. Twenty-five seems to be the magic number for repetitions, and many people use beads or knots in a piece of string to help count them out, although fingers will do just as well. There are striking similarities here to Christians counting out their prayers on rosary beads and the Greek tradition of worry beads.

Speaking affirmations out loud harnesses a lot of energy – in much the same way as prayers or mantras call on the energy of all the times they have been spoken in the past.

Like most other measures for change, the effectiveness of these PTRs seems to depend on the energy and commitment with which they are used. I have known people work with affirmations for an assortment of things from finding or selling houses to improving skin conditions – all with great success.

The metre or rhythm of the affirmation is also important, so a simple, tuneful and specific saying works best – 'Today's the day I begin to recover' or 'Now I am starting to make myself better', rather than 'I am ready to start to improve the condition of my health'. If the affirmation can rhyme, so much the better – it seems to be a short-cut to activating the subconscious. Good examples are: 'Now is the time my ... is fine'; 'Today's the day my ...'s gone away'; 'Now it's revealed my ... is healed'.

Visualising the completed wish is a powerful aid which works very well alongside affirmations. The more ways you can find to help make something happen, the more techniques to focus you on your desire, the more time spent imaging it as reality, the more likely it is to occur.

Affirmations are a good way of formalising the tick-a-tape or unspoken thoughts that are always flowing through our heads. This background noise of criticism, praise or general chit-chat is ignored by us most of the time – we regard it rather like an old familiar friend whose story is known by us only too well. Whether this voice is a pessimistic, blaming, conscience/ devil, or a rich, rewarding, encouraging angel, its energy can be harnessed and used to focus consciously on what we need in our lives. Imagine if all that muttering were to be transformed into clear words of active encouragement, focusing on confirming what we believe or hope to be true. This is the real power of affirmations.

Affirmations can be used whenever you have a spare moment during the day, although it is a good idea to set aside a specific time as well. Spending ten minutes at the beginning or end of each day on a variety of techniques that will make your vision a reality is a good habit to get into. Beyond that, any time you may make will reaffirm your commitment to achieving your goal. Many psychics, counsellors and therapists will help clients devise their own affirmations as a positive way of continuing the work done in the session, and to encourage reliance on their own unique power to make happen the life that they choose.

Further reading

Milton Erickson, *My Voice Will Go With You*, Norton, USA.

Piero Ferrucci, *What We May Be*, Crucible Thorsons Publishing, 1982.

Kenneth Meadows, *The Medicine Way*, Element Books, 1990.

ANALYSIS

Self-analysis

Analysis is a term we are now all familiar with. Strictly speaking it refers to psychoanalysis, a distinct form of therapy based on the teachings of Freud, or analytical psychology which is based on the teachings of Jung. The work of analysis is based on a detailed exploration within a highly formalised structure of the analysand's (or client's) history of events and emotions from birth to the present day. Freud's beliefs were based on his own personal experiences and those of the many people he saw in his practice. He believed that early conflicts were at the root of most individual distress, and did much pioneering work in the field of human sexuality. The fundamental belief in Freudian analysis is that the person's psyche is completely determined by the events of the first five years of life. Jung expanded upon these early ideas and focused more on the concept of archetypes or universal images and consciousness and their positive effects.

Entering analysis requires a strong commitment and can involve up to five sessions each week for many years. Many analysts prefer the analysand to lie on a couch, and will sit just out of their line of vision. This is what has given rise to the term 'doing the couch trip'.

Self-analysis however, is something that is free and available to

16

to everyone who chooses it. I see this useful tool rather as an exercise in de-coding. Often, things that occur in our lives and our own information about these events seem to be clouded from consciousness or expressed through symbols.

We can all, for example, learn to understand our dreams through the symbols we use in them. You don't need to be a shaman or clairvoyant to build your own vocabulary of symbols. Once you learn the meaning of a word, that is the word you use to express an idea or to identify something; symbols are non-verbal 'words', and once learned (or interpreted) will be used in the same way.

Analysing dreams is an effective way to 'keep tabs on' our true feelings. Keeping a dream diary is a lovely way to honour the unspoken communication we have with ourselves, and interpreting those dreams cements that relationship between our conscious selves and what seems to be going on underneath the surface.

> Thinking about symbols and what they mean to you is a good place to start. You may like to make a list – a house, a tulip, a landscape, an ocean, whatever you feel is relevant – and write down what ideas or images come to mind. You may image a cottage tucked into the hillside with smoke curling out of the chimney when you think of a house. Does it feel as cosy as it looks? Perhaps this is a symbol of security; if so, feelings of insecurity might be pictured as the cottage in ruins, or with a storm raging and no chimney smoke, or maybe as a city tower block, its complete opposite. These are only suggestions – most people discover their own silent vocabulary to be a wonderfully rich and worthwhile surprise, and it will most certainly be unique to them.

Analysis of our conscious actions and motivations can often be affected by distancing ourselves from them. Simple measures such as writing down the situation in need of clarification in a letter and posting it to yourself can be remarkably revealing.

Listing the pros and cons of a decision can also yield unexpected results and important insights. One patient of mine agonised for weeks over whether to move house. She eventually made a list of all the reasons why she should, all the benefits to be gained, and all her objections. She ended up with two pages full of good reasons to move and only six reasons not to, but one of those was the immensely powerful 'I don't want to'. She was then able to see the decision in a much clearer light – as being between what made logical sense but betrayed her feelings and what she didn't want to do but might be seen as a good idea. She had loaded down the logical side because, for her, one ounce of feeling equalled at least three kilos of logic in any equation. (She didn't move house.)

One of my teachers, Betty Balcombe, uses a triangle to help clarify situations. Draw a triangle on a sheet of paper and write your problem in the centre. On the left of the triangle list the events which lead to the dilemma, track back to when and where the problem began. On the right side, list what needs to be done, what help is needed, who needs to be seen or what extra information is needed. This gives you a clear picture of the past, the present and what can be done to help. When all the possible action has been dealt with, the choice becomes much clearer.

Self-analysis is really self-regulation and can lead to a more complete or holistic understanding of ourselves and our actions. It enables us to use more of our mental capacity, and to integrate it with the rest of our experience.

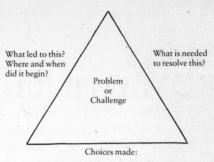

One method for problem solving

Finding out more

Association of Jungian Analysts
3–7 Eton Avenue
South Hampstead
London NW3
Tel: 071 794 8711

Society of Analytical Psychology
1 Daleham Gardens
Swiss Cottage
London NW3 5BY
Tel: 071 435 7696

Further reading

Betty Balcombe, *As I See It*, Balcombe Books, 1988.

Eric Berne MD, *A Layman's Guide to Psychiatry and Psycho-analysis*, Penguin Books, 1968.

Strephon Kaplan-Williams, *Transforming Childhood – A Handbook for Personal Growth*, Element Books, 1990.

Kenneth Meadows, *The Medicine Way*, Element Books, 1990.
Dr Brian Roet, *All in the Mind? think yourself better*, Optima, 1987.

AROMATHERAPY

This is any treatment using the aromatic oils obtained from a variety of plants for their medicinal properties.

These 'essential oils' are extracted from the leaves, stems, roots, or any part of the plant in a variety of ways; using water extraction, heat treatment, or oil basing. Once extracted, they can be used in their pure and extremely potent form, or diluted using a carrier oil.

The pure oils can be taken internally in drop form, and used to treat a variety of conditions – it is important that only the purest oils are used in this way, and they should never be taken without the advice and monitoring of a qualified and experienced practitioner. This method of treatment is used extensively on the Continent, and is gaining popularity in the UK.

The most common way of using the oils is in dilute form, in a base or carrier oil. These can then be added to bath water or further diluted in oil and used in aromatherapy massage.

The essential properties of the plant oils impart different qualities – some sedative, like basil; others stimulating, like rosemary; or balancing, like lavender. There are essential oils to calm the nerves, stimulate digestion and help depression for instance. In all cases, it is the aroma of the oil which is said to be one of the most active properties. Smell is the quickest route to the brain, and the smell association area in the brain is next to the part concerned with memory. This explains the evocative nature of aromas – how they can conjure up memories and feelings from times long gone. This also accounts for many of the mood-changing qualities of aromatherapy treatments.

Aromatherapists will most usually use massage as their form of treatment, although it is worth checking that this is the case with individual practitioners. Almost all the oils can be used safely at home, although they should never be taken internally without the advice and monitoring of a qualified and experienced practitioner. The pure oils should never be applied directly to the skin in case burning should occur.

At home, they can be added to bath water, as a therapeutic addition to a foot bath, for self-massage and, either dispersed in water or burned, as a room scent. The powerful effect of these oils should not be underestimated, and, as a general rule, add no more than three drops to bath water or similar and no more than five drops to a saucer of carrier oil for massage.

The drops of oil can be added to running bath water and keeping the bathroom door closed ensures that the aroma in the steam remains in the room and can be inhaled while you soak. There are some bath oils on the market which contain essential oils in a dilute form, so much more can be added. It is important to check the label to make sure you don't add too much of a pure oil.

There is a variety of oil burners available which act as room fragrancers, although they do need to be watched lest they burn dry. Two drops of oil added to a vase or bowl of water will fragrance a room, particularly in warm weather or if the bowl is placed near a source of heat. Another good idea is to place a few drops on a dry cloth and wipe over any light bulbs; as the bulb heats up the fragrance is slowly released into the room.

Essential oils may be diluted and worn as a perfume, or mixed with an emulsifier and added to a machine wash (or to the final rinse of a hand wash) to delicately fragrance clothes or upholstery.

On visiting an aromatherapist who uses massage, you might expect the initial appointment to last anything from an hour to one and three-quarter hours. This is so that there will be time for you to get to know each other and for the practitioner to take a brief history from you. You may be asked for any relevant medical information and also more general questions about your feelings and emotions. Certainly your mood that day and any particular aches and pains you might have will assist the practitioner in selecting the appropriate oils. Once the history is taken you will be asked to undress and lie on the massage couch. As a general rule, some people leave on their underwear, and those who are comfortable in undressing completely do so. The practitioner will be quite used to working with people in various states of undress, so you can follow your own feelings as to what feels best.

The aromatherapist should be able to answer any questions you may have about the treatment and will also take your lead on whether to talk or not – some people find they like to be quiet while they are being massaged, others prefer to talk a little.

At the end of the treatment you will have some time to rest and gather yourself before getting dressed again. The practitioner may then suggest some oils for you to add to your bath water, to use as a room scent, or whatever is appropriate. This is also the time when you can arrange another appointment. Subsequent visits are likely to be shorter because the practitioner will already have your history or notes and will usually just want an update on how you are feeling and what your reaction was to the last treatment.

It is advisable to wear casual clothes, or to take a change of clothes with you because the carrier oils used for the massage can stain some synthetic mix fabrics like poly-cotton quite badly. Some clinics will have a shower facility, but it is nice to let the oils continue to be absorbed through your skin and to carry the aroma for a while after the treatment.

Aromatherapists can be found at many alternative health-care clinics, and at some gyms, fitness centres and hair and beauty salons. Some work from home, and you may be lucky enough to find one who will visit your own home, bringing with them a massage couch and a selection of essential oils. Some aromatherapists advertise in the Yellow Pages and in health food shops and similar outlets, but, as with any practitioner, a personal recommendation is by far the best guide.

There are dozens of oils currently on the market. Some, like jasmine, are very expensive because the amount of oil obtained from each plant is so small, and it needs to be handled very carefully during processing; then of course there are the costs of shipping and packaging. Other plants, like rosemary, grow in many more parts of the world and yield their oil more easily. Essential oil of rosemary is relatively inexpensive.

Here is a small selection of essential oils that would form a good basic kit for home use. Care must always be taken during pregnancy (when some oils are contra-indicated), and aromatherapy oils should not be used without the advice and monitoring of a healthcare practitioner.

Oil	Properties	Home uses
Clary sage	Warming, soothing	Good for the chest – use in steam inhalations and to massage locally
Eucalyptus	Respiratory cleanser	In steam inhalations – to clear sinuses place one drop on a handkerchief or pillow

Frankincense	Rejuvenating	Comforting in states of anxiety. Use in a steam inhalation to deepen breathing, in massage or baths
Geranium	Refreshing, balancing	Good for stabilising the emotions. Added to other oils in massage, in baths or as a room freshener
Howood	Woody, evocative	Pelvic decongestant – add to a footbath or bath; room scent
Jasmine	Anti-depressant, mood enhancer	In massage, baths; good for scenting clothes and rooms
Juniper	Kidney tonic, toxin eliminator	Stimulating in baths and foot baths and for local massage
Lavender	Balancing, relaxing, immune stimulator	Universal balancer – its action is normalising, analgesic and antiseptic. One drop added to water relieves pain of insect bites and burns
Peppermint	Refreshing, cooling, digestive aid	Cooling and invigorating. Good for digestive disorders and nausea. Effective insect repellent

Rosemary	Stimulating, cleansing antiseptic	Strengthening and invigorating; clears mental dullness and aids circulation
Sandalwood	Particularly good for mature skins, aromatic	Sweet and woody; often used to evoke a meditative atmosphere. Useful for anxiety and nervous tension. Has an affinity with the kidneys so can gently support them
Tea tree	Anti-fungal, anti-viral	Use on spots, bites, sores and athlete's foot. Useful for thrush. Dab on to cold sores three times a day for fast relief
Ylang ylang	Soothing, sensual, exotic	A reputed aphrodisiac – powerful, sensual stimulant

Finding out more

Aromatherapy Associates
68 Maltings Place
Bagleys Lane
Fulham
London SW6 2BY
Tel: 071 731 8129

Association of Tisserand Aromatherapy
65 Church Road
Hove
East Sussex BN3 2BD
Tel: 0273 772479

Micheline Arcier Aromatherapy
7 William Street
London SW1X 9HL
Tel: 071 235 3545

Further reading

Patricia Davis, Aromatherapy, An A–Z, C.W. Daniel Company, 1988.

Daniele Ryman, *The Aromatherapy Handbook*, Century Publishing, 1984.

BAREFOOT THERAPIES

Reflexology · Metamorphic Technique

Barefoot therapy has a prominent place in natural healthcare. We all know how much good feeling can be generated from this small area of the body – simply freeing your feet from shoes and stockings or socks at the end of the day brings relief to most people. Letting feet breathe, unhampered by synthetic fibres or the confinement of footwear has important health applications too.

Many foot problems stem from lack of air, or misshapen shoes. Fungal conditions such as athlete's foot thrive in moist, warm conditions, and allowing the feet to breathe is an important part of taking care of them. People often find that the natural shape of their feet bears little resemblance to the shape of the shoes that house them for up to eighteen hours each day, so little wonder that corns, bunions and other hard spots develop. You can check this for yourself with two sheets of paper and a pen: stand with one foot on a sheet of paper and your weight evenly distributed on both legs. Bend down and draw around the shape of your foot, or ask somebody to do it for you. Then put on your shoes and repeat the process, and compare the results. The differences are usually most striking with women who wear high-heeled shoes.

Taking early morning dew walks on a patch of clean grass;

or paddling in the cool waters of a stream on a hot day, or amongst the waves along a beach, can bring enormous pleasure and directly stimulate this important part of our bodies. Learning to explore with feet; defining textures and rediscovering how much they can do are all such worthwhile activities. We spend so much time using them for propulsion and to bear our weight that it is easy to forget how sensitive feet can be.

There are disabled individuals who write, paint and do much more with their feet. I knew a woman who trained her toes to move up and down independently of one another and thought she was quite remarkable in this, until I heard of another woman who had done the same, and another – it seems all it takes is time and concentration. It seems only right that this capable, sensitive and useful part of the body should be given more care. Bringing feet into contact with fresh air and walking barefoot for some time each day allows the muscles of the foot to be exercised and is very grounding; really putting us in touch with the world we walk on. I feel, too, that this warms some distant genetic memory in the tremendous feelings of well-being that it can generate. Our distant forebears spent much time barefoot, only using a protective covering as they became more adept, and only then for crossing difficult terrain.

In many societies and groups today footwear is removed as a sign of respect and at times of personal reflection. In Moslem societies, for example, people take off their shoes when entering a mosque and shoes are often removed in order to meditate. A growing number of people do not wear shoes in their homes at all.

In our search for total health and well-being, we cannot ignore the promise and the joy that freeing our feet can provide. There are two therapies that treat the feet; or that aim to treat the whole body through contact with the feet: reflexology and metamorphic technique.

Reflexology is a science that deals with the principle that there are reflexes in the feet which relate to all parts of the body. With the client seated, or lying back with their head raised, the reflexologist works using tiny pressure movements over both surfaces of the bare foot and around the ankle. The movements follow a map which details the parts of the body and the corresponding reflex point situated on each foot. The spine reflex, for example, lies along the inside line of the foot stretching from the base of the big toe down towards the heel; and the solar plexus is just below the ball of the foot, in line with the second toe. The liver, spleen and other organs are all represented along with areas of the body like the head and neck (found in the toes).

Reflexologists aim to effect beneficial change on an overall basis, as well as to stimulate or relieve specific areas or organs. They can feel which areas are in need of support through the changing texture of the feet as they work on them. Very often, the client will also feel some areas to be more sensitive than others, and may be aware of the physical links – experiencing stomach gurgling while the digestive system is worked on for instance, or a change in breathing as the sinus area is cleared. An experienced practitioner will be able to notice the changes through subsequent treatments and chart the client's progress.

I love my feet being touched or massaged and respond very well to it, but even those without such leanings normally find reflexology treatments to be very relaxing. The touch should be firm enough not to tickle, yet not so hard as to be painful – although occasionally an area will be very sensitive, and practitioners will often take this as an indication of some form of imbalance in the body part to which that spot relates. They will sometimes work on this area on the other foot, and then return to the site of discomfort where the original sensitivity will usually have decreased.

A short course of treatments, perhaps four or six, is most

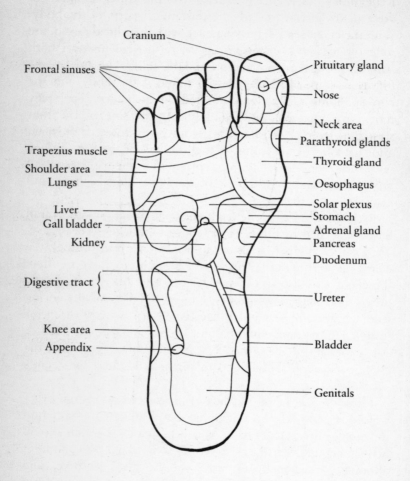

Cranium

Frontal sinuses

Pituitary gland

Nose

Neck area

Parathyroid glands

Trapezius muscle

Thyroid gland

Shoulder area

Lungs

Oesophagus

Liver

Solar plexus

Gall bladder

Stomach

Adrenal gland

Kidney

Pancreas

Duodenum

Digestive tract {

Ureter

Knee area

Appendix

Bladder

Genitals

Right foot

Reflexology Tables

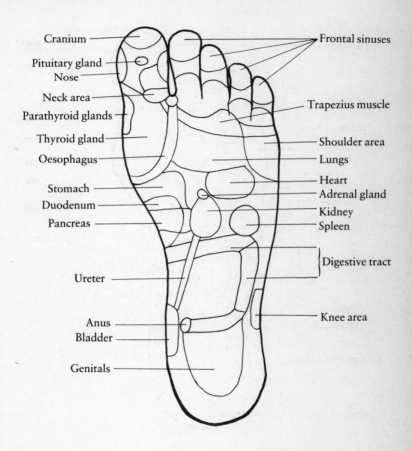

Cranium

Pituitary gland

Nose

Neck area

Parathyroid glands

Thyroid gland

Oesophagus

Stomach

Duodenum

Pancreas

Ureter

Anus

Bladder

Genitals

Frontal sinuses

Trapezius muscle

Shoulder area

Lungs

Heart

Adrenal gland

Kidney

Spleen

Digestive tract

Knee area

Left foot

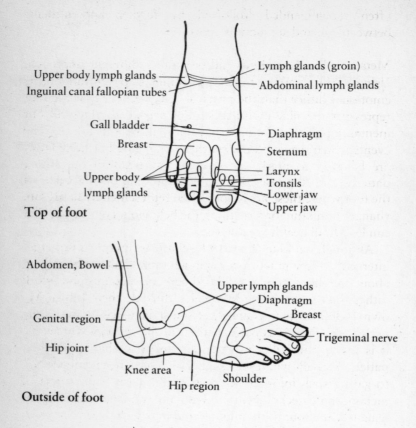

Top of foot

Upper body lymph glands
Inguinal canal fallopian tubes

Lymph glands (groin)
Abdominal lymph glands

Gall bladder
Breast

Diaphragm
Sternum

Upper body
lymph glands

Larynx
Tonsils
Lower jaw
Upper jaw

Outside of foot

Abdomen, Bowel

Upper lymph glands
Diaphragm
Breast

Genital region

Trigeminal nerve

Hip joint

Knee area

Hip region

Shoulder

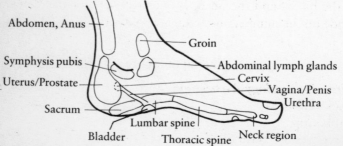

Inside of foot

Abdomen, Anus

Groin

Symphysis pubis

Abdominal lymph glands
Cervix

Uterus/Prostate

Vagina/Penis
Urethra

Sacrum

Bladder

Lumbar spine

Thoracic spine

Neck region

often recommended, followed by further appointments between one and six months apart.

Metamorphic Technique takes a quite different approach. Using a light, feathery touch, practitioners concentrate on the emotional rather than the physical. They believe that the foot represents the nine-month gestation period in which all our mental, physical, emotional and spiritual patterns are set. The events which regulated our mother's changing hormone levels are believed to mark our growth and establish our future patterns and responses. By gently smoothing out the areas of the foot where these are found (often represented by hard skin, changes in texture or structure), the behaviours or stresses that can lead to ill health are relieved.

Although working at such a level, the technique is not at all interactive – the practitioner is much more likely to be talking about unrelated topics or the theory of metamorphic work rather than whatever they perceive through their hands. My own feeling is that change can most beneficially and truly occur with conscious participation. In the spirit of wholeness, it is the responsibility of the practitioner to share with their patient or client whatever insights may have been gained. Not to garner such information, or to withhold it is an aspect of metamorphic technique that I do not understand. Sessions usually last about thirty minutes and may include similar work on the hands and the head. It is usually left for the client to decide on the number and frequency of visits.

Finding out more

British Reflexology Association
Monks Orchard
Whitbourne
Worcestershire WR6 5RB
Tel: 0886 21207

British School of Reflexology
92 Sheering Road
Old Harlow
Essex CM17 0JW
Tel: 0279 29060

International Institute of Reflexology
PO Box 12462
St Petersburg
Florida 33733
USA
Tel: (813) 343 4811

Metamorphic Association
New Cross Natural Therapy Centre
67 Ritherdon Road
London SW17 8QE
Tel: 081 672 5951

Further reading

Mildred Carter, *Helping Yourself with Foot Reflexology*, Parker Publishing, West Nyack, New York, 1969.

Avi Grinberg, *Holistic Reflexology*, Thorsons, 1990.

Anya Gore, *Reflexology*, Optima, 1990.

Gaston Saint-Pierre and Debbie Boater, *The Metamorphic Technique: Principles and Practice*, Element Books, 1988.

BODY FORMS

Yoga · T'ai Chi · Qi Gong · Ki Aikido

There are many practices which it would be difficult to describe solely as exercise or martial art or energetic movement, although they may encompass some or all of these descriptions. The body forms provide a way of practising the integration of body and mind, and strengthen their connection.

Yoga is often treated as an exercise in the West, although its origins are as a complete discipline – one covering the physical, spiritual and mental planes – and this is how it continues to be experienced in the East.

As a system of exercise the gentle stretching can be beneficial for certain body types, although the need for a highly qualified and experienced teacher cannot be over-emphasised. Ideally, the physical positions should be achieved through a gentle easing and relaxing of the muscles, and careful monitoring is required to ensure correct posture. I have treated a number of patients who needed osteopathic care after doing a yoga class. These were all people who had joined a large group (twenty or more), and had moved into advanced yoga positions too early in their tuition. Being told to 'just go as far as you can' is often taken as an instruction to push oneself into an extreme position. Without exception, these individuals attended a weekly class and did not practise by themselves between lessons. Their injuries could all have been avoided by proper assessment, guidance and instruction by their teachers, and an understanding of the need to approach yoga gently.

As a complete discipline, yoga is said to be tremendously empowering and transformational, uniting body, mind and spirit in a single focus designed to provide a method for living and a tool for lifestyle change. With this focus, the practice of the yoga positions (or asanas) would include specific breathing exercises (pranayama), deep relaxation techniques and meditation skills, although there are also sexual, karmic and lifestyle yoga practices.

T'ai Chi does not ostensibly offer such a comprehensive range of skills; it is a form of ritualised movement which nevertheless is said to work on the physical and spiritual planes. To watch an accomplished practitioner is a great joy; there is an elegance about them and an ethereal quality seldom seen in other Forms. They appear as if moving through water, as weight is slowly shifted from one foot to the other while the body and the arms work through a variety of slow circular movements. With the body grounded (bent knees assist in lowering the centre of gravity) the aim is that the sequence of movements once learned can flow on their own; one does not 'do' T'ai Chi, rather one *is* the movement. The Chi (Chinese term for vital energy) is encouraged to move freely; an enormously pleasurable and profoundly beneficial experience.

Often called moving meditation, T'ai Chi is practised by Buddhist monks and nuns. The movements are excellent exercise for the body and their gentle nature aids contemplation and relaxation. Based loosely on Taoist principles of balance and harmony, T'ai Chi is practised all over China and can often be witnessed in parks and town squares as people practise 'the form' during work breaks and lunch hours.

The form may be short or long and there are different styles, but all flow with the same grace and ease of movement. T'ai Chi classes will often start with simple warm-ups before going on to practise the prescribed movements. Often a strengthening exercise of **Qi Gong** will be taught – these are a range of postures and stretches which strengthen the vital energy and encourage an easing of the meridians or energy pathways which network the body. These can also be practised on their own as a system of physical healthcare.

Ki Aikido is a Japanese martial art which focuses on the spiritual development and awareness of the individual.

Physical strength is not necessary in Ki Aikido, because the emphasis is on finding ways to use the aggressor's own force against them. Students practise using great concentration on their own energetic state, and learning techniques which will harness the momentum of an attack for use as defence.

Students develop an awareness of 'one point'; the physical centre of gravity that is often called hara. This is a point just below the navel and its energetic importance is as the site where the physical and spiritual energies in the body meet. One technique is called 'keeping weight underside'. This is to maintain the sense of being grounded and is a way of consciously maintaining physical relaxation. If you hold out your arm and try to exert strength to keep it in position, it will tire and become harder to hold, therefore potentially easier for another to move. If you concentrate on holding it in a relaxed way, aware of your own centre (hara) and the presence of gravity (keeping the weight on the underside) it is harder for somebody else to move it.

Ki Aikido is taught in classes of anything up to thirty students and they progress through a grading system, signified by the wearing of coloured belts. The highest grade is a black belt. Although Ki Aikido is essentially an art of self-defence, the practitioner's aim is to develop sufficient skill and awareness to make it unnecessary to engage in any form of physical combat. Ki is the Japanese word for life force, 'ai' means union and 'do' means path or way. The word then, and the practice, incorporates the individual's vital energy into a way of living.

Finding out more

Iyengar Yoga Institute
233a Randolph Avenue
London W9 1NL
Tel: 071 624 3080

British T'ai Chi Ch'uan Association and London T'ai Chi Academy
7 Upper Wimpole Street
London W1M 7TD
Tel: 071 935 8444

School of T'ai Chi Ch'uan
Centre for Healing
5 Tavistock Place
London WC1H 9HH
Tel: 071 459 0764

British Ki Aikido Association
c/o The Secretary
48 Oakshott Court
Polygon Road
London NW1 1ST
Tel: 071 281 0877

Community Health Foundation (East West Centre)
188 Old Street
London EC1V 9BP
Tel: 071 251 4076

Martial Arts Commission
First Floor
Broadway House
15–16 Deptford Broadway
London SE8 4PE
Tel: 081 691 8711

Further Reading

Chungliang Al Huang, *Embrace Tiger, Return to Mountain*, Celestial Arts, USA.

Man-chi'ing Cheng, *Cheng Tzu's Thirteen Chapters on T'ai Chi Ch'uan*, North Atlantic Books, Berkeley, 1985.

Silva Mira and Shyam Mehta, *Yoga, The Iyengar Way*, Dorling Kindersley, 1990.

Jon Pearson, *An Introduction to Aikido*, Optima, 1991.
Alan Peek, *An Introduction to T'ai Chi*, Optima, 1990.
Bob Smith and Linda Boudreau Smith, *Yoga For A New Age*, Smith Productions, 1988.

John Stevens, *Aikido The Way of Harmony*, Shambhala Books.

Chögyan Trungpa, *Shambhala: The Sacred Path of the Warrior*, Shambhala Books, 1984.

BODYWORK

Many physical therapists and healers call themselves body-workers. This phrase embraces a range of therapies and most often bodyworkers use a synthesis of different techniques they have developed for themselves. In the course of their training, and with the wide variety of available workshops, few physical practitioners stick solely to one particular set of skills.

My own interpretation is of work that is both physically moving and also involves some form of psycho-emotional content – either a counselling aspect or, more generally, a body/mind philosophy of which the client is made aware.

Bodywork essentially encompasses two main types of therapy – structural bodywork, which is concerned with achieving individual change by focusing on altering or correcting physical imbalances and allowing these to influence the whole person; and body-orientated psychotherapy. These latter techniques place greater emphasis on the body as container or manifestation of personal impulses, and seek to release emotional and mental blocks from their physical sitings.

Rolfing was devised by Ida Rolf as a way of completely rebalancing the body by realigning any asymmetry. Rolfers work using their hands, elbows or knees to apply deep pressure to the muscles and release them from any habitual or ineffective positioning.

The work involves ten sessions, usually lasting one hour or slightly longer each. Rolfers will begin by assessing the body from all perspectives – sideways, backwards, etc. – to get an overall picture of how all the structural elements stack together. Standing in their underwear, the patient or 'rolfee' will then be photographed. This allows a good before and after comparison to be made, and the rolfee may have copies of both shots.

Rolfing sessions progress through the body, working on one specific area each time. There is a degree of pain involved as the rolfer reaches down deeply into under-used or tired muscles, and rolfees are encouraged to express the pain, so yelling and groaning often accompany a session. The effects can be really dramatic – as the before and after photos will confirm, and most people comment on the mental or emotional changes they experience during the ten sessions.

Rolfing has lead on to the establishing of several other forms of structurally aligning bodywork, most notably hellerwork, aston patterning and primal integration.

Hellerwork takes a gentler approach to release adhesion in the muscle tissue, and the emphasis with this type of work is on verbally processing the emotions and thoughts which come up during the bodywork. Movement education to increase self-awareness is also a facet of this therapy.

Aston patterning relies more on movement to achieve optimal structural integrity and is again much gentler on the body than rolfing. **Postural Integration** unites the rolfing concept with the ideas of Wilhelm Reich, that a degree of tightness or body 'armour' is a necessary product of developmental and everyday psychological stresses. This allows a more psychotherapeutic element to be brought into the sessions, and enables the mental and emotional releases stemming from the bodywork to be addressed within a treatment.

Bioenergetics is the most established Reichian-based therapy. Reich's theories explore the healing capabilities of the body which he maintained was driven by instinctive or sexual 'life energies'. He repeatedly asserted the fundamental role of individual sexual energy in continued good health, and encountered much resistance for so doing. A few years before his death in 1957, Reich was imprisoned ostensibly for ignoring an injunction against his research work, and this is where he died of a heart attack after having all of his books and papers burned.

Dr Alexander Lowen and others refined Reich's basic therapeutic techniques to form Bioenergetics, a system that directly addresses any repressed desires and lack of vibrancy or vitality to unite mind, body and energetic process.

Sessions include the holding of a number of physical exercises or postures which, alongside breathing techniques, allow stagnant energy to be mobilised or released. The client or patient is encouraged to express the emotions that come up as energy flows through their body. The work alternates between perceiving and releasing muscular–emotional blocks, and talking about what is happening, to gain insights as to the nature of the blocks.

Grounding and breathing exercises begin each session to focus the client in their body, and these along with many of the other exercises can be practised alone, in between sessions, to continue the work.

Grounding is about feeling as if you live in your whole body, not just in your head. It is about 'knowing where you stand' and 'having your feet on the ground' – embodying your life.

Sessions usually last for one hour or slightly longer, and may be booked as frequently as the client desires. Many people like to book a few initial sessions quite close together and vary the frequency according to the nature of the issues they are dealing with.

One excellent grounding exercise is to bend forward as if to touch your toes. Move your weight onto the balls of your feet and let your upper body relax completely and just hang down towards the floor. Continuous breathing helps intensify the experience – this is just as it sounds; breathing deeply but without leaving any gaps between breaths. With the weight moved forward on to the balls of the feet, the hamstring muscles at the back of the thighs are stretched tight and may well begin to shudder or shake. The idea then is to slightly exaggerate the shaking, allowing it to increase as much as it needs to, and keep breathing. Sometimes the shaking subsides spontaneously, at other times it may lead to strong memories entering the mind or feelings welling up.

The advantage of doing this in a session is that whatever feelings or ideas come up can be expressed and then processed and understood; placed in the context of your life. When doing this alone, it is a good idea to process in some way whatever material comes up – write it down, draw it, talk to someone about it, or find some way of working with it. Your body will have just released a precious piece of information and it needs to be recognised and honoured.

It might be that nothing happens beyond a little quivering in the muscles, which spontaneously subsides – when this is the case there is a resulting feeling of great relaxation in the legs, and people have often said it lets them feel 'as though they really reach to the floor'.

In dipping into the reservoir of feelings and memories that the body holds, all these forms of bodywork serve to remind us of the rich connections between all parts of ourselves.

Finding out more

Rolf Institute
80 Clifton Hill
London NW8 0JT
Tel: 071 328 9026

Hellerwork
The Peak Club
Hyatt Carlton Tower
London SW1X 9PY
Tel: 071 243 0132

The Aston Training Centre
PO Box 544
Mill Valley
California 94941
USA
Tel: (702) 831 8228

British Institute for Bioenergetic Analysis
22 Fitzjohns Avenue
London NW3
Tel: 071 435 1079

Institute of Bioenergetic Medicine
103 North Road
Parkstone
Poole
Dorset BH14 0LU
Tel: 0202 733762

Open Centre
188 Old Street
London EC1V 9BP
Tel: 071 549 9583

Further reading

Don Johnson, *The Protean Body: A Rolfer's View of Human Flexibility*, Harper Colophon, 1977.

Alexander Lowen, *Bioenergetics*, Penguin, 1979.

Alexander Lowen and Leslie Lowen, *The Vibrant Way to Health: A Manual of Bioenergetic Exercises*, Harper and Row, 1977.

Ida P. Rolf, *Rolfing: the Integration of Human Structures*, Dennis-Landman, 1977.

CLAY THERAPY

Used extensively by many naturopaths, clay may be taken internally in liquid form or used externally in a pack applied to the skin. It is composed of a layer of silica oxide around a layer of aluminium oxide with a mixture of minerals that will determine its consistency and colour, e.g. magnesium, iron and calcium. The strong attractive qualities of clay make it particularly helpful in speeding up the elimination of toxins and poisons from the body.

Mixed into a paste with a high quality vegetable oil, it can be applied to the skin as a soothing agent and is used to help relieve a variety of irritated skin conditions. The addition of a drop or two of tea tree essential oil makes a very effective treatment for fungal conditions like athlete's foot, and adding lavender essential oil helps to soothe the skin even further.

The paste can be applied as a poultice over a very small area – to draw out a boil, for instance – or as a body pack, covering up to 70 per cent of the skin surface for more widespread conditions. In acute situations, e.g. a widespread allergic reaction of the skin, the paste can be applied before bed and rinsed away the following morning. This can help alleviate any sleeplessness and night-time scratching as well as improving the condition of the skin.

Taken internally as a drink, clay is especially useful in light cases of heavy metal or fungal poisoning. Many people take it on a regular basis for its qualities as a blood cleanser and its role in increasing the oxygen content of the blood. Although its aluminium content does not leak into the system, its long-term internal use is not recommended in old age, pregnancy, pre-conceptual care, lactation or in immune-compromised individuals.

Clay can also be used as a cleansing agent in place of soap or shampoo, and this is especially useful in the presence of any contact allergies and for irritated skin. An effective cleanser, the clay does not challenge normal skin pH.

For the use of clay in modelling and as a medium of expression, see Creative Therapies.

Further reading

Harry Lindlahr, *Natural Therapeutics*, C.W. Daniel, 1975.

Ross Trattler ND DO, *Better Health Through Natural Healing*, Thorsons, 1987.

COUNSELLING

Counselling can take many forms depending upon the counsellor's training and the individual's reasons for seeking this type of support. Most usually it will address a particular issue or difficulty, and last for a relatively short period of time. These are the main differences between counselling and the psychotherapies, which generally require a longer-term commitment to working in a much wider context. (See Talking Therapies). To muddy this distinction, however, there is also psychological or psychotherapeutic counselling, which works at a deep level with the individual's own process.

People often seek out a counsellor for advice or support in much the same way that the advice of elders or wise men and women would be sought in other societies. The North American Indians have a tradition of seeking this wisdom from the spirit of their ancestors, or from the Shamans which are common in this and other cultures.

Counselling for specific situations is clearly labelled – **Health Counselling** or **Bereavement Counselling** for example, where people with these difficulties may find help. The initial session is a time for both people to see whether they want to work with the other, and also when it is important to determine precisely what is needed and what the counsellor can provide. It may be that practical advice is sought, or, as is often the case, that what is really wanted is someone who will listen, without judging.

An enormous benefit provided by a counsellor is their objectivity – they may have, and voice, their own opinions, but there is no existing relationship; you begin your work with a counsellor without any previous history, and in the sure knowledge that whatever is discussed in a session will be completely confidential.

This discretion enables people to explore things fully in a safe environment before integrating it into their lives. It may be that the counsellor is used as a sounding board, to try out new ways of relating; or as an important source of support during times of change.

The techniques used in a session will depend on the counsellor's training as well as the individual's reasons in seeking out this form of help. Two basic types of skills are employed – directive or active counselling and a more receptive approach. The latter builds on the work of Carl Rogers who developed a style known as **Client-centred Therapy**. He maintained that the only frame of reference that could be of any use to a client would be one which they built themselves. In practice, this means that the focus of the work is in defining and clarifying the client's own understanding and resources. Counsellors working in this way will mirror the client; on the simplest level often repeating or simply rephrasing what they hear and offering it back to the client.

This is a very good technique for use in times of distress, when the individual is often unable to take in advice or new ideas and will respond best to a validation of their own feelings. It is also extremely useful for encouraging confidence in one's own thoughts and ideas and in increasing the client's feelings of self-esteem.

More directive approaches include those working within a

particular framework – such as **psychological astrologers**. They have information to impart as well as the offer of a new perspective or framework within which to view both the current situation and developmental factors. **Psychic counsellors** also work actively, translating what they perceive of or in a person in an effort to give them as much pertinent information, and therefore as great a choice, as possible. Visits to both psychological astrologers and psychic counsellors are likely to be on an irregular basis, or even as 'one-offs'.

Although the basics of all counselling sessions are the same – the client and the practitioner both talk to each other; sometimes over a desk, sometimes on a sofa in a sitting-room type situation – that is really where the similarity ends. It is important to establish what you are looking for as early as possible in your search for somebody to work with. It is also necessary to be prepared to have appointments with a variety of different counsellors before finally deciding on one.

Sometimes you will establish a rapport immediately, or have a positive gut feeling that this is the person you want to work with. In order for the sessions to be as productive as possible, you will need to find someone who you feel you can trust and whom you feel understands you. If particular things are important to you in your choice of counsellor, perhaps sexual orientation or political awareness, then it is appropriate to ask this of them in the same way as you might enquire as to their experience in the field, or any areas of special interest that they might have.

Sessions usually last for between fifty minutes and an hour, and their frequency will usually be agreed during the first or second visit. In the case of couples counselling, where both partners are seeking assistance together, this may take longer to establish. In some instances it may be appropriate to agree to a fixed number of appointments, perhaps four or six, and then to reassess the situation. This provides an opportunity to get on and tackle a specific area of difficulty at the same time as allowing the counselling relationship to develop.

Counsellors usually take their clients by referral from other practitioners, although some also advertise in specialist journals and locally at Citizens' Advice Bureaux, etc. This usually happens when a counsellor is just beginning their work, and is seeking to build a strong client base.

A good place to find a counsellor is through the training colleges, who keep registers of their graduates. Those offering long courses will sometimes encourage students to begin work before they qualify; they then work for a reduced fee and should get good supervision from their course tutors.

Details of specific counsellors – for debt, bereavement, etc. – can be found at most local libraries and CAB offices.

Finding out more

The British Association for Counselling
37A Sheep Street
Rugby
Warwickshire CV21 3BX
Tel: 0788 78328/9

Centre for Alternative Education and Research
Rosemerryn
Lamorna
Penzance
Cornwall TR19 6BN
Tel: 0736 810530

Centre for Counselling and Psychotherapy Information
21 Lancaster Road
Notting Hill
London W11 1QL
Tel: 071 221 3215

Faculty of Astrological Studies
396 Caledonia Road
London N1
Tel: 071 700 3556

***Relate** (formerly Marriage Guidance Council)*
Herbert Gray College
Little Church Street
Rugby
Warwickshire CV21 3AP
Tel: 0788 73241
Local addresses in the telephone directory.

Further reading

W. Dryden *et al* (editors), *Handbook of Counselling in Great Britain*, Routledge, 1989.

Susan Lendrum and Gabrielle Syme, *Gift of Tears – A Practical Approach to Loss and Bereavement Counselling*, Routledge, 1992.

S. Quilliam and I. Grove-Stephenson, *The Counselling Handbook*, Thorsons, 1990.

Rosamond Richardson, *Talking About Bereavement*, Optima, 1991.

CRANIAL THERAPY

Cranio-sacral therapy and cranial osteopathy are exquisitely gentle yet profoundly effective methods for treating the whole body and effecting structural change.

Although called cranial, the techniques can be used throughout the body and often involve some form of direct contact with the patient's energy field. The release of holding patterns within the body may also allow emotions to surface and become conscious. The gentle nature of the work makes it particularly helpful in the treatment of newborn babies, older people, those in pain, and in any situations where more physically based treatments would be inappropriate.

Developed in the early 1900s by the pioneering work of an American osteopath, William G. Sutherland, this 'new' therapy is in fact steeped in ancient tradition and healing lore. Some of the earliest pictorial records of healing show a simple 'laying on of hands' and written evidence tells of 'the art of listening'. This is the essence of cranial work. The practitioner uses the hands to listen to or feel the intrinsic movement patterns of the person; and employs simple techniques to magnify them or to lead the body into releasing and re-balancing itself.

Sutherland investigated the structural links between different areas of the body. He developed a theory that the bones of the skull could, by their positioning, affect and be affected by other areas of the body. To substantiate this, he began his work by developing a type of American football helmet with chunks of movable padding. He experimented on himself by using the helmet to limit the movement of specific cranial bones, and carefully noted his physical and emotional responses. He soon discovered that areas as distant as his toes could be affected by the immobilisation of these bones, and charted a host of emotional reactions also. His wife wrote a touching account of what it was like living with him during this time – in particular not knowing what sort of a person he would be from one day to the next: bad-tempered and irritable, or back to normal.

Sutherland then went on to work with the soft tissues and fascial arrangements of the body, and developed his theories further to include an appreciation of the body's subtle structural integrity and movement patterns. He noted that all the bones of the body display an almost imperceptible movement, and discovered the key sites where interruption of such movements or blockages could be relieved.

This work was further developed by Dr Randolph Stone, who expanded some of Sutherland's concepts, and in the 1960s and 1970s by Dr John Upledger who synthesised the techniques into a full-body approach.

The prime source of this inner motion is the process of cerebro-spinal fluid production and reabsorption. CSF is a viscous, jelly-like substance produced by the brain which provides protection for it and the spinal cord. It bathes and envelops the system, encased by the meninges and the bony protection of the bones of the head and spine. If the brain were a precious gift, CSF would be the packing material, the meninges a cling-film coating to hold it all together and the bones would be the presentation box.

The movement of the CSF can be perceived through an experienced touch, and its rhythms and patterns of motion yield a wealth of information as to the condition of the whole body. Other body movements can also be felt in this way – the sway of all the bones in response to breathing; the waves of peristalsis moving through the gut; even the minute, fluid motions of the organs themselves. Connecting with these rhythms and bringing them to the patient's awareness is often enough in itself to effect change.

Treatment is a deeply relaxing experience, enabling the patient to still their conscious mind and place their attention on their own inner resources. Feeling only the weight, or even gentler touch, of the therapist's hands, they can perceive subtle inner changes. Becoming aware of alterations in internal pressure, movements and releases of energy is often accompanied by changes in breathing patterns (the breath may slow or become deeper) or stomach gurgles – a good sign of relaxation.

People will often be aware of what is occurring in one part of their body while the therapist's hands are placed some distance away. This is due to the continuity of fluids and fascias (a sort of inner skin for the muscles and organs) throughout the body; everything is connected. Most often, as the treatment progresses, the patient becomes more and more relaxed and the therapist's touch almost imperceptible. People often describe their feelings as those of actually being inside their own bodies, or of being in touch with their own energetic state; losing the sense of being separated from the world by their skin. This can lead to mystical, religious or 'peak' experiences.

Cranio-sacral therapy is often used as a technique for personal growth because of the great understanding and insights it can provide. It is tremendously effective on a physical level too; in its gentleness it can be used for structural change when the body is in too much pain to allow an osteopathic adjustment, and its depth allows it to access long-term or deep-seated physical difficulties.

There are a number of bones in the head – in a baby these

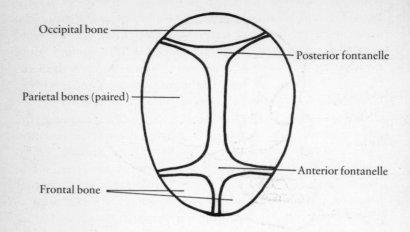

Occipital bone

Posterior fontanelle

Parietal bones (paired)

Anterior fontanelle

Frontal bone

The foetal skull seen from above

are separate to allow some contraction as they move through the birth canal. The fontanelles, which are evident at birth, are the potential spaces for the bones should they be needed during the journey through the birth canal. As the baby gets older, these fontanelles disappear from sight as the bones grow closer together. The joins between the bones, however, remain potentially mobile throughout life.

Some health difficulties can be traced back to the birth process and the first few months of life, and the release of any obstructions felt between the bones of the skull can be tremendously beneficial. This is particularly so if forceps or suction techniques were used during the birth. It is becoming increasingly common for cranio-sacral therapists or cranial osteopaths to be present at a birth or to treat both mother and baby immediately afterwards.

Most cranial workers are osteopaths who have studied cranio-sacral techniques as post-graduates, although some people take the route from another form of healing. The advantage of an osteopathic training is the thorough know-

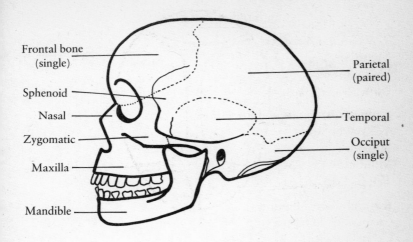

Frontal bone
(single)

Sphenoid

Nasal

Zygomatic

Maxilla

Mandible

Parietal
(paired)

Temporal

Occiput
(single)

Mobile bones of adult skull, side view

ledge of anatomy and physiology, and an understanding of the laws of mechanics as applied to the body. They will also have a greater knowledge of general pathology. All of these can be learned, however, and those coming to the work without manipulative concepts may be more open to its subtler aspects.

Treatments usually take place with the patient lying on a treatment couch, and fully relaxed, although some techniques need the patient to be seated. Sessions last an hour, on average, and there will often be time after the treatment to discuss the therapist's findings and the patient's perceptions. This is particularly important if the patient has experienced the work at a deep level, as they may need to talk about their experience and any implications on an emotional or spiritual level. Sometimes, of course, the treatment is almost exclusively physical, in which case the time may be used for postural advice or ongoing care details.

Finding out more

The Cranial Academy
Meridian
Idaho 83642
USA

Cranial Osteopathic Association
478 Baker Street
Enfield
Middlesex EN1 3QS
Tel: 081 367 5561

Karuna Core Therapies
Curtisknowle House
Curtisknowle
near Totnes
Devon TQ7 7JX
Tel: 054 882 583

The Upledger Institute
11211 Prosperity Farms Road
Palk Beach Gardens
Florida 33410
USA
Tel: (800) 223 5880

Further Reading

Harold Magoun, *Osteopathy in the Cranial Field*, Journal Printing Co, Missouri,

William Sutherland, *The Cranial Bowl*, Free Press Company and Journal Printing Company, Missouri.

Adah Sutherland, *With Thinking Fingers*, Cranial Academy, Kansas City

Johnn E. Upledger, DO FAAO and John D. Vredovoogd MFA, *Cranio-sacral Therapy*, Eastland Press, Seattle, 1983.

CREATIVE THERAPIES

Drama · Art · Music · Voice · Toning · Dance

There are many creative forms that can have therapeutic applications. Drama, art, play and dance therapy are available amongst others, and many can form part of a supportive everyday routine. Although there are professionals in all these subjects, they can certainly yield benefits when practised individually.

Any sort of creative pursuit can be a fulfilling part of our lives. We all have creative energy, and it is there to be used. The variety of channels for this is enormous – some people pour it into their work, others separate it completely. Whichever you choose, it is important to acknowledge its role in your life as a fundamental part of living life to the full. Whether you express that creative energy biologically, through bearing children; professionally, in the choice of a career in the creative fields; in your leisure time, or in your very private life is a matter of personal choice.

You don't need to join a group to express your creativity – drawing or painting your feelings, or putting them into dance is something you can do at home or wherever you are; when the mood takes you or for a specific period to introduce the practice of creative expression into your life. Drama and play are not ostensibly solitary pursuits although if you have ever watched children at play, totally immersed in a private imagining, you have an idea of what is possible. On this level, the adult alternative would be constructive fantasy.

Taking some time each day or at least each week to enrich your creative talents while leaving aside any work ethic can be wonderfully beneficial. Letting go of the need to be in control, or to behave in a certain, specified way is incredibly liberating and can be lots of fun too.

Drama therapy or psychodrama is a popular choice of creative pursuit, with a therapeutic bent. Taking place in groups of anything up to thirty people (although around twelve is usually the norm), it involves the other participants to act out the roles of characters in your own life, and then you in turn may play the part of someone important to them. Under the direction of the therapist, this provides the opportunity not only to figure out individual situations in an active and realistic way, it also draws on the intuition and feelings of the other group members. A variety of resolutions to any theme can be explored and experienced and this dynamic form of acting out can quickly lead to an understanding of what feels right.

Sometimes our true feelings can become buried underneath the obligations and restrictions that come to bear in real life situations, and this opportunity for make-believe can yield tremendous insights. After each enactment, time is given to reflection on the true feelings that emerged.

An intimacy and feelings of safety are soon generated by groups that work in this way, and to aid these meetings may start with the therapist suggesting some group games. These are most often mental and physical exercises aimed at increasing the trust between group members and act as a gentle warming up period for the work to follow. Most people find these very enjoyable and just as beneficial as what happens in the rest of the class.

Art therapy seeks to explore and release feelings through their expression in drawing, painting or modelling. These can then be interpreted using the artist's own symbology and/or the insights of the therapist. This direct means of expression by-passes the cognitive or censoring part of the brain and can reveal valuable clues as to the artist's own self as well as providing an exciting new way to tackle involved or difficult matters. Art therapy can be explored on its own or as part of many psychotherapeutic models. Or, you can do it yourself, without analysing it, for the great pleasure it can provide.

Although often taking place in groups, art therapists will also offer individual sessions. Many people find the group situations offer more security, especially if they are not experienced with this medium of expression, because it is sometimes difficult to get started and the presence of others relieves them of any feelings of responsibility to 'perform' or draw or paint to order. This is also a 'safer' place to start – allowing time to feel easier with the chosen means of expression before exploring more deeply that which has actually been expressed. The contribution and insights of the other group members can also be extremely helpful.

Different classes will take a variety of approaches, some using the time to focus on a theme which can then be illustrated, others using the class time in a more analytical way by spending time on discussing work done prior to meeting.

Music as therapy is used a lot by people with mental and physical disability, providing a valuable means of expression and stimulus. Its use has become more widespread to meet the universal need for new avenues of expression and ways to understand the inner feelings which are sometimes difficult to validate. Pouring emotion into music is what makes it good – allows it to resonate with something within the listener.

The mood changing effects of music are known to us all. Its evocative nature marks it as an effective means of communication and it has many uses within the community; unifying groups and creating atmospheres more effectively than just about anything else. Gentle, soft sounds and easy melodies can aid relaxation and meditation; faster, more rhythmic music can help with more energetic activities.

Using music as therapy may be the perfect way to begin to develop creativity, or a safe form of channelling emotions, or an energetic release. There are many ways of using this medium – concentrating on rhythm and its hypnotic effects, for example, as in drumming, or on performance. Most usually, this therapeutic use of music is active; involving playing an instrument or singing although it may also involve listening to music.

People are often surprised to find how well they can evoke a feeling with an instrument. If someone were asked to play a violin their initial reaction is likely to be refusal. Being asked to be *loud* on a violin, however, presents few problems. Once this confidence is felt, it becomes easier to let the feelings through and from there comes the ability to acknowledge and begin to understand and accept them.

Using one's **voice** can be a wonderfully healing experience. Whether it is through singing or chanting or toning, the feeling of 'playing one's own instrument' is deeply rewarding. A

Toning is a seemingly simple technique – the vibration of a note or sound is said to resonate with a variety of different body areas and motivational energies. Singing the note can clear the energy in that area of life and help resolve conflicts and blocks. You can try it for yourself by singing any sound and changing the pitch to different notes – some will sound clearer or sweeter than others. If you find a note that sounds tinny or unclear and keep singing it, you will hear and feel the change as it becomes fuller.

perfect method for creative expression, singing can teach us much about our own abilities and motivations, and help with our own flow of energy throughout the body. So many people think that they can't sing or hold a tune, and while a performance singer requires special training, learning to express oneself through voice can unblock massive creative potential for personal growth on many levels.

Music and voice therapy are usually conducted (!) in groups, although most therapists also offer individual sessions where deeper, more analytical work can take place.

Dance has always been an important part of human experience – as a means of personal expression, for connecting with the environment, bonding within the community, and as ritual. Dance therapy encourages individuals to explore the body through movement. Various styles have developed; some concentrating on the therapeutic aspects of what our body positions and movements say about our inner feelings; others focusing on the development of creative expression. Working in groups, sometimes with music, sometimes not, the dancers can allow their bodies to flow and move in a free, unstructured way.

The teacher may point out areas of restricted movement by mirroring them, or by inviting the dancer to find words or another way of demonstrating the feeling behind their action. Classes usually begin with some warming up exercises before going on to expand individual movement sections.

This is a wonderful choice of therapy for those wanting to get more in touch with their physicality, and also for those who feel that they intellectualise too much. Moving freely and expressing our feelings thereby is something we all knew how to do in childhood, and dance is an excellent way of recapturing that childlike freedom. There is real magic to be experienced when you give yourself to the dance and a sense of wonder the first time your body moves knowingly, without conscious planning.

The physical work-out involved in a class and the experience of the freedom to move creatively strengthens the links between mind and body. This can have positive spin-offs – one being the wonderful side effect of encouraging greater flexibility in a variety of other areas of life. Participants often experience the benefits of classes overflowing into their everyday lives. Once a confidence is gained, it becomes easier to express creativity and physicality in other ways, and in a host of other situations.

Finding out more

5 to Midnight
5 Bittaford Terrace
Bittaford
South Devon PL21 0DX
Tel: 0752 894 675

British Association of Art Therapists
11a Richmond Road
Brighton BN2 3RL

Dance Education and Training
5 Tavistock Place
London WC1
Tel: 071 388 5770

Dancing on the Path
39A Glangarry Road
London SE22
Tel:081 693 6953

Holwell Centre for Psychodrama and Sociodrama
East Down
Barnstaple
Devon
Tel:027 282 267

Inner Sound and Voice Workshops
c/o Gillian McGregor
Garden Flat
9 Yonge Park
Highbury
London N4 3MU
Tel: 071 607 5819

Laban School for Movement and Dance
Goldsmiths College
Laurie Grove
London SE14
Tel: 081 692 4070

Living Art Training
11 Stowe Road
Ravenscourt Park
London W12 8QB
Tel: 081 749 0874

Open Centre
188 Old Street
London EC1V 9BP
Tel: 071 549 9583

Playspace
Short Course Unit
Polytechnic of Central London
35 Marylebone Road
London NW1 5LS
Tel: 071 486 5811 ext. 465

Playworld
2 Melrose Gardens
New Malden
Surrey
Tel: 081 949 5498

Person-Centred Art Therapy Centre
17 Cranborne Gardens
London NW11 0HN
Tel: 081 455 8570

Further reading

H. Blatner, *Acting In*, Springer, 1976.

T. Dalley, *Art As Therapy*, Routledge & Kegan Paul.

J. Fox, *The Essential Moreno* (drama therapy), Springer, 1987.

P. Holmes and M. Karp, *Psychodrama: Inspiration and Technique*, Routledge.

Keith Johnstone, *Impro (Improvisation and the Theatre)*, Methuen, 1989.

M. Keyes, *Journey: Art as Therapy*, Open Court, 1984.

R. Laban, *The Mastery of Movement*, Northcote House, 1980.

Gabrielle Roth, *Maps to Ecstasy*, New World Library, USA.

DETOXIFICATION

This is something that our bodies should be doing all the time. The elimination of toxins through a variety of routes enables the body to function properly and ensures good health. Many medical philosophies maintain that it is this process of clearing out the body that facilitates good health, and that disease is a natural result of a failure to eliminate or a break down of the body's eliminative routes.

A clear example of this is the bowel. Irritable bowel conditions, cancers and a host of other gut disturbances are most common in societies with a high intake of refined foods. When these are eaten at the expense of the natural roughage which is to be found in fruits and vegetables, the walls of the colon can become clogged and ineffective. This means a lowering in the rate of absorption of nutrients from the foods we eat, but can also result in some substances remaining in the gut for years!

There are a number of avenues available for such elimination. The liver does much of the work of filtering substances within the body and these can be expelled through the work of the kidneys, in urine; through the skin, by perspiration; the lungs and mucous membranes; and the bowel. The efficient functioning of all routes is necessary to full health. This can easily be seen when a period of constipation is accompanied by spots or pimples appearing on the skin, or in the obvious fluid retention and bloating that can occur the morning after a larger than usual alcohol intake.

The body is continually producing substances which need to be expelled – every muscle activity, chemical process and stage of growth leads to an amount of unnecessary by-products or debris. Each hormonal, emotional and energetic response creates substances which the body needs to be rid of. And most of the chemicals we ingest through the foods we eat, the air we breathe and the substances we contact have no place in our system.

There are a number of measures we can take to ensure that our eliminative routes and organs are functioning as well as they can. Dry skin brushing (see Skincare) and good personal hygiene aid skin function, and drinking adequate amounts of fresh, clean water helps the kidneys work well. Diet is one of the most effective ways of clearing the bowel and can also allow the whole body a time to cleanse. Eating foods that are as close as possible to their natural state releases a large amount of energy for use within the body. When we simplify the job of digestion, we liberate the huge amounts of energy that are usually used to discern, process and progress food-stuffs. This energy can then be used to concentrate on detoxification and any other healing work that is needed.

Nature provides us with obvious times to detoxify. Each change of season marks a transition from one form of behaviour to another, the range of foods which is naturally, locally available to us alters, as do the ways we spend our time, and the body changes its rate of metabolism.

This transition period is a time to use diet to support the whole system – making life as simple as possible so that the body's own vitality can control its resources and do whatever work is necessary.

If we look at the foods which are naturally available, we can see some times of year being more abundant than others. Harvest time in autumn has traditionally been a time of feasting; late winter, before the first spring shoots appear, a time of fast. Women have their own inner 'seasons' as they move through their monthly cycle.

There are detox diets which last for a month or more, and these give the body an opportunity for a thorough cleanse as well as providing good support to the immune system. Spending just a few days on simple foods can be useful too, or one day each week on some form of mono-diet. This is a very individual thing and all people respond differently – eating only apples or pears on one day each week might fit brilliantly into one person's schedule, yet be impossible for another.

A simple diet of brown rice, steamed vegetables and lots of salad gives the body a wonderful rest and allows much background maintenance and healing work to be done. Following this for three days at a time will serve as a rejuvenating filip for the whole system. If done during the summer months, more emphasis can be placed on the salad part of the meal, indeed some people may wish to eat only raw food. In the winter, the addition of some cayenne pepper and ginger will help keep the body warm.

Food combining is another tool that suits some people excellently, others not at all. Separating protein from carbo-hydrates can make things simpler for some people's digestion and this can be done in a small way by eating the protein part of any meal first, the carbohydrate at the end. (In this scheme of food combining, vegetables with the exception of potatoes are considered neutral.) Others need to separate protein meals from carbohydrate meals altogether.

During the warmer months, spending a few days eating only

raw food is an excellent way to boost the body's eliminative powers. During winter, the addition of cooked brown rice and steamed vegetables makes for a good clear out (in the colder weather you need the warmth from the cooked food). These mini-diets can be repeated once a month or, for a more sustained effect, spend one day each week on some form of fast.

There are different types of fast – from a dry fast in which no food or drink is taken at all, to a mono-diet in which only one type of food is eaten. Dry fasting should never be attempted without the advice and monitoring of an experienced practitioner, but a day each week spent eating only apples, pears or drinking freshly-made vegetable or fruit juices can be highly beneficial. It is inadvisable to follow a strict cleansing diet for more than three days without professional advice.

When detoxifying or following a mono-diet for a day or longer it is important to keep warm and remember to drink lots of fresh, clean water. Any amount of exercise you do will reinforce the work of the diet and help liberate toxins. Energy levels may fluctuate, however, and it is common to feel lighter and more energetic, but not to have the usual amount of staying power – people often find they tire more easily. Sleep patterns may also alter – people usually find they need less sleep and wake feeling fresher, but may need to rest more than usual. All of this is because the extra energy liberated by making digestion less of a task is being used internally to mobilise the body's defences, pep up the metabolism and, of course, to eliminate.

Some of the first benefits to become obvious are a clear skin, which can be seen almost to glow; a brightness around the eyes; and a feeling of lightness which translates into the way we move – often noticed as a spring in the step or a more confident posture. On longer-term diets (three days or more) the speed at which the body mobilises toxins can for a time supersede the capability of the eliminative routes. This can lead to a period of experiencing mild headaches, some spots on the skin (particularly on the face) and feelings of lethargy. This never lasts for more than a day, and can be so mild as to pass almost unnoticed; it all depends on the individual level of health and vitality.

Most of these measures can be undertaken individually, but if assistance or support is required, any naturopath should be able to monitor your progress and make individual suggestions. Fasting and detoxifying are an important part of the naturopathic system of healthcare.

Biologically, we are still 'hunter-gatherers'; our systems are used to periods of fasting or low food intake, and eating large amounts of food *every* day is a relatively new idea. Regular detoxification allows our bodies time for rest and renewal within our busy schedules and is a positive aid to preventative healthcare.

Finding out more

Incorporated Society of Registered Naturopaths
1 Albermarle Road
The Mount
York
YO2 1EN

Further reading

Belinda Grant, *The Detox Diet Book*, Optima, 1991.

Doris Grant and Jean Joice, *Food Combining for Health*, Thorsons, 1984.

Henry Lindlahr, *Natural Therapeutics*, C.W. Daniel, 1975.

DIET THERAPY

The foods we eat provide essential building blocks for continued good health. Dietary therapy covers the range and types of food eaten each day as well as specific diets for individual purposes, e.g. to treat a condition or to lose or put on weight.

We are what we eat – literally! Our bodies are constantly rebuilding – everything from our skin to our bones has its own cycle of growth and elimination, and the foods we eat provide the material for that growth. A good diet is one of the most important steps we can take towards continued good health and prevention of disease.

There are many factors to consider when looking at the foods we eat – among others their condition and freshness, the nutrients they contain and benefits they can provide, how and when they are eaten, and their chemical components.

It seems obvious that our food should be in good condition – we would not choose to eat a rotting apple or a piece of mouldy bread. We tend to tell a lot about the quality of a food from its appearance, and in the past this was a good indication of its state. Nowadays, however, this is often far from the truth. The many processes that even fresh fruit and vegetables are exposed to is daunting and this is before we think about processed, canned or freeze-dried produce.

Much of the fruit we buy has been chemically treated,

waxed or even irradiated. The average apple has undergone twenty-three chemical processes by the time it reaches the shop shelves. Admittedly, some of these are repeat sprayings of fungicides, pesticides or fertilisers, but it still makes for a complicated chemical cocktail. So much for 'an apple a day ...'. It frightens me when I hear that the pesticides that are banned from our drinking water because of the health hazards they pose are the same pesticides that are routinely used on much of the food we eat.

Organically grown foods are the only viable alternative to slowly poisoning ourselves. On the whole they taste better and the labelling is honest – when you buy an organic carrot, that's all you are getting; not a carrot plus an assortment of poisonous or noxious substances whose long-term effects on humans are unknown.

The market for organics is growing all the time, which means there are now more and more products available and the prices are coming down. Organic produce is still much more expensive than chemically grown foods. A variety of organically reared animals, milk and cheeses are appearing in the shops, along with a growing selection of fruits and vegetables. With careful shopping, up to 70 per cent of any diet can now be organic, and the difference will be felt straightaway.

How we handle food is another important consideration for ongoing health. The closer a food is to its natural state, the more beneficial it is likely to be. A large amount of raw food eaten each day ensures a good supply of nutrients and facilitates peristalsis; the way food is moved through the gut. Raw fruit and vegetables contains cellulose, a natural form of fibre that moves easily through the digestive system cleansing it as it goes. The fresher the plant, the more vitamins and minerals it will contain. Vitamins fall into two categories – water-soluble and fat-soluble. The water soluble vitamins are lost as soon as they are cooked, so even in winter raw foods form a valuable part of the diet.

The way that food is cooked can conserve or destroy its valuable nutrients. Steaming is better than boiling, for example, because it avoids the best part of the food being thrown down the sink with the water. Different cooking methods are more appropriate to certain seasons, too: long, slow, oven cooking which conserves the goodness and energy of food is perfect for the winter months; quicker methods like stir-frying seem in tune with nature as spring comes.

These are just some of the factors a naturopathic dietary therapist will consider when working out an individual eating plan with their patient. Obviously, personal likes and dislikes are important, but so too is recognising that these are sometimes governed by the response of jaded taste buds or allergies. Our taste buds can adapt to large amounts of salt and chemical flavour enchancers, but once these are removed from the diet our sense of taste can recover giving us a clear picture of the subtler flavours and tastes we really enjoy.

Ordinary table salt should not in fact be on *any* table, but moved to the bathroom (see page 188). There is enough natural sodium in the foods we eat without adding extra to any cooked meal. In the West we use salt far too liberally as a flavour enhancer, and, like all flavour enhancers, our palates quickly adapt to want more and more of it. It is often added to cooking as well as to prepared food, and is present in most tinned and processed foods. Once removed from the diet, the natural taste of food can shine through and the amazing recovery powers of your taste buds will delight you in their rediscovered sensitivity. Too much salt added to the diet can lead to fluid retention and can compound high blood pressure and heart problems.

Allergies pose a complicated challenge to naturopaths. Sometimes the foods we have an allergy to are those we crave, or that are a staple, regular part of daily meals. The connections between dairy intake (milk, cheese, butter) and mucous conditions is well documented – chestiness, sinus conditions and continuous cold-type symptoms respond well to the removal of dairy foods from the diet. We still tend to think of milk as a nutritious, health-giving drink, though – governments promote it and it is still provided in some schools. Wheat has a proven implication in arthritic complaints, yet this has a regular place in most diets. Where necessary, then, a practitioner may recommend abstinence from some everyday foods for a period of time.

Other allergies may be less obvious; I have an allergy to the oxylate family (tomatoes, rhubarb, spinach and sorrel are the main culprits) although sometimes just one member of a family can cause difficulties. The problems caused by an allergy can range from severe headaches to a general lack of energy or an aggravation of other conditions.

Genetic factors are important here, too – a growing number of Europeans are experiencing mild potato allergies; a direct legacy of the vegetable's prominent position in the diet over the last 100 years. Those with Mediterranean forebears may exhibit sensitivities to olives – they and their oil being widely used throughout the region. Or if a parent had a strong allergic response to a certain substance, then that may appear as a sensitivity in their child.

However, allergies to the artificial additives and chemical compounds with which foods are adulterated are by far the most common.

Naturopathic dietary therapists will have two main concerns – to encourage a healthy and varied basic diet and to deal with any specific health difficulties. They can suggest particular diets to help with a number of complaints, from arthritis to migraines, or may propose changes in diet from season to season.

Keeping a diet diary is a useful way of identifying any possible aggravants and of obtaining an overview of our eating habits. You may be asked to keep one for a few days prior to your first visit to a naturopath.

DIET ANALYSIS SHEET

Day:
Breakfast:

Drinks:

Lunch:

Snacks:

Dinner:
Physical feelings after eating:
Overall energy levels:
Emotions:
Notes:

Remember to note when meals are eaten, and in what environment – whether you are relaxed or stressed; business or at home; in a restaurant or home cooked, etc. These factors can yield as much information about your reaction to what you eat as the foods themselves.

Keeping a diet diary for a few weeks can highlight possible allergens, but is also very telling about how balanced your basic diet is.

This and the information you give in the consultation will help to build a clear picture of your current nutritional status. Many therapists will suggest a course of vitamin and/or mineral supplements for you to take, alongside the changes in your diet.

You may also be advised to add some foods – it's not all about taking foods away. The use of foods for their healing and curative qualities is another important aspect of naturopathy. Beetroot is a great liver tonic and can help with clearing the system; alfalfa stimulates and supports the spleen; cabbage is useful in cleansing the skin; and there are many other foods which support and help the body in similar ways.

I am currently seeing an increasing number of people who need to add some animal protein to their diets. Disgraceful methods of animal production are encouraging more and more people to give up eating animal flesh altogether. Some do very well and are much healthier this way, but I believe that some people do need animal protein in their diet in order to stay healthy. Organic rearing and humane killing methods mean that dignity can be restored to the animals bred for human consumption. I can understand the dilemma, but feel that the important moral concerns need to be balanced with our search for full health. It is important to stick to our principles, but not if the price is our own health and well-being. If the objection to eating meat is the immoral treatment of animals that robs them and us of dignity, then sound, caring, responsible animal farming is certainly a step in the right direction.

Dietary therapy is concerned not just with the foods themselves, but with the context in which they are eaten, the background, the season and the condition of the foods themselves. All these factors are as important as the individual's constitutional needs. Lifestyle makes a difference, as does a person's inherent vitality and their ability to eliminate unwanted substances from the body. Whether their circulation is good, if they have a sedentary job, at what time of year they feel their best and a variety of other factors will all help to determine individual requirements.

Treatment is often an ongoing process, with sessions increasing in regularity as health considerations change. Most often, an initial course of appointments will be followed up by visits at the change of each season and then an annual checkup.

There are also dietary therapists or nutritional counsellors who do not have a naturopathic training. Their main considerations will tend to be the nutritional values of the foods themselves, without placing them in the wider context of healthcare that naturopathy provides. These therapists often rely on supplementing the diet with vitamin, mineral and glandular formulations to achieve fuller health.

Finding out more

British Naturopathic Association
6 Netherhall Gardens
London NW3 5RR
Tel: 071 435 6464

Dietary Therapy Society
34 Priory Gardens
London N6 5QU
Tel: 081 341 7260

Eating Disorders Association
Sackville Place
44–48 Magdalen Place
Norwich NR3 1JE
Tel: 0603 621414 (9am–4pm weekdays)

Green Farm Nutrition Centre
Burwash Common
East Sussex TN19 7LX
Tel: 0435 882482

Incorporated Society of British Naturopaths
Kingston
The Coach House
293 Gilmerton Road
Edinburgh EH16 5UQ
Tel: 031 664 3435

Nutrition Society
10 Cambridge Court
210 Shepherds Bush Road
London W6 7NJ
Tel: 071 602 0228

Further reading

Carol Bowen, *A–Z of Health Foods*, Hamlyn Publishing Group, 1979.

Dr Stephen Davies and Dr Alan Stewart, *Nutritional Medicine*, Pan, 1987.

Henry Lindlahr, *Natural Therapeutics Vol III – Dietetics*, C.W. Daniel, 1975.

Ross Trattler, ND DO, *Better Health Through Natural Healing*, Thorsons, 1985.

ENERGY WORK

Shiatsu · Jin Shen Do · Polarity Therapy · Reiki

All matter is composed of energy and there is a range of therapies that work with the energy of an individual as it manifests in and around their body. There are many different approaches to this work and healers work with this energy in a variety of ways.

There are those who follow a system of energy channels in the body corresponding to the acupuncture meridians. Some, using **Shiatsu**, will apply a constant pressure to points they call tsubos which cover the whole body. This pressure is usually applied with the fingers and hands directly onto the skin, although the practitioner's feet and elbows may also be used on heavier parts of the body like the hamstring muscles at the back of the legs.

Most usually, the practitioner begins by deciding whether there is an overall condition of insufficient energy (kyo) or unexpressed energy (jitsu), and the treatment will vary according to this judgement – either dispersing any pent-up energy or helping the body to conserve it. Some practitioners will take the pulses, or use tongue or facial diagnosis to help reach this important decision, while others rely on their psychic or intuitive skill and experience.

Once the body has begun to balance in this way, more attention can be paid to specific points along the particular meridians or pathways that the practitioner senses to be in need of attention.

The pressure used in Shiatsu usually feels very positive, although sometimes it may build up just to the point of pain. An experienced practitioner will be able to read the body well enough never to exceed this and cross the threshold to cause actual pain.

Shiatsu originated in Japan and is still used there and in China as a form of primary healthcare, regular treatments being seen to be an active preventative measure. Dependent upon your individual needs, you may expect to feel either deeply relaxed or pleasantly energised after a treatment. Sessions usually last for about an hour, with the initial consultation lasting longer to enable a health history and other important information to be exchanged. As this sort of work is so energy-reliant, it will vary considerably between individual practitioners and so it is important to find one with whom you feel a good energetic connection.

There is a charming story of a man in Japan who tried to find somebody to give him Shiatsu. He 'phoned for a visiting practitioner and settled down to await his arrival. The Shiatsu Master who usually ran this service was unable to attend him and a recently qualified student of his went along instead. So, the newly qualified practitioner arrived and began his work. After only four or five minutes the man stopped him saying, 'I asked for Shiatsu, not a student'. Despite the practitioner's assurances that his qualifications were indeed sound the man explained that 'Your hands are busy – that is no way to give Shiatsu'.

This illustrates the quality of the work involved. The person giving the Shiatsu treatment must have 'empty hands' – hands that are totally receptive and responsive to the body on which they are working.

The perfect training for this is in a refinement or cousin of Shiatsu called **Jin Shen Do**. Many people maintain that whether the work they chose to pursue is actively physical, as in Shiatsu, or subtler in nature, as in Jin Shen Do and similar disciplines, the understanding and ability to sense that is cultivated in these latter practices is a prerequisite for beginning treatments.

Jin Shen Do practitioners use a similar map to those who practise Shiatsu, but rarely use pressure on the tsubos or body points, preferring a holding or slightly pulling touch. This is altogether different from a Shiatsu treatment, feeling much less physical and seeming to reach a deeper level within the individual. More time may be spent on diagnosing a person's condition, and again this may be through light touch or psychic assessment and the practitioner will then seek to encourage the flow of energy through the body with these gentle contacts. The whole body is not usually covered in the same way as in Shiatsu; rather the Jin Shen Do practitioner will elect a smaller number of points and hold each for a longer period of time. This form of treatment has been likened to the ancient Chinese 'Art of Listening', in that work is done in a meditative state and the feeling afterwards is that one's body, with all its silent stories, has been truly heard.

Both forms of treatment require the patient to be at least partly undressed, and although Jin Shen Do may be performed with the patient lying on a couch, the more active Shiatsu usually takes place on the floor. As part of a session may involve use of the practitioner's full weight on the patient's body, a wide floor space is required. This usually consists of a thin, padded mattress similar to a futon which is then covered, so the body is fully supported.

Polarity Therapy uses another understanding of anatomy, seeing the central energy source, or core of the person, as neutral, and all points beyond that as being either positively or negatively charged. Polarity therapists maintain that the soles of the feet, for instance, are negative poles and the head is a positive pole, the palm of the left hand having a negative charge, the palm of the right a positive charge. Practitioners use their hands to balance these varying energy states by placing them on the body at prescribed locations.

Reiki or Radiance Technique is part of a full system of healthcare that includes dietary and exercise aspects, but in its bodywork is ostensibly similar to the other forms mentioned here, requiring gentle, caring touch. The focus with Reiki, though, is on allowing Universal Energy into the individual, or helping them to expand so that they may receive it.

Treatments with all these forms of therapy usually take place with the patient lying down in order that they may be as relaxed as possible. The work can be carried out however the patient is placed, but whilst lying down they will be comfortable and can feel quite secure – it is easier to close one's eyes and relax more fully in this position. It also allows the practitioner an easy contact with most of the patient's body – an important point, because nothing is less conducive to relaxation than to have somebody fumbling to reach the inside of your arm, or having to move you around too much.

Most treatments take place in a reflective or meditative atmosphere and there is no rush. As important as the treatment itself is the time taken immediately afterwards to reflect on what has occurred, and to re-orientate oneself ready for the rest of the day. If the work has been deep and effective, then there may well be thoughts or feelings that you may wish to discuss with the practitioner. If feeling deeply relaxed then you will want to take some time to 'wake up' again and get back in touch with your current reality. Many people liken their reaction to some of these treatments as having been in a dream-like state – like that experienced just before sleeping.

All these different styles concentrate on working with the individual's own energy, and the energetic exchange with the practitioner or therapist. That this is the focus of the work marks these as distinct from other therapies, but it is worth remembering that all contact, whether physical or not, involves some form of energetic communication. An awareness of this is often what makes the difference – marking a really good reflexologist, masseuse or manipulative therapist. In any form of bodywork, a sense of, and respect for, the individual's energy is most important, although an exchange does also occur in non-contact therapies.

There are healers and psychics who use off-the-body work, involving some movements of the practitioner's hands over the body at a distance of a few inches. They are still working with the individual's own energy field which extends a distance beyond the physical body and forms the aura. Some also use absent healing, when the practitioner can be any distance away (see Healing).

It is possible to feel moved by, attracted to or irritated by someone's energy even though you are not in contact – most of us have experienced this – or feeling a strong response to somebody before you've even spoken. A skilled practitioner can use their perception of this to add insights to any counselling session, or to aid diagnosis. Developing this awareness for yourself can enrich self-growth and responsibility, and add a quality to communication with others.

Finding out more

British School of Shiatsu-Do
188 Old Street
London EC1V 9BP
Tel: 071 251 0831

Shiatsu Society
14 Oakdene Road
Redhill
Surrey RH1 6BT
Tel: 0737 767896

Jin Shen Do Foundation
PO Box 1097
Felton
California 95018
USA
Tel: (408) 338 9454

Polarity Therapy Association UK
11 The Lea
Allesley Park
Coventry CV5 9HY
Tel: 0203 670847

Radiance Education Unlimited (Reiki)
PO Box 1013
London NW3 3LW
Tel: 071 586 2980

Further reading

Betty Balcombe, *As I see It*, Balcombe Books, 1988.

Gerald Jampoulski, *Love Is Letting go of Fear*, Foundation for Inner Peace, 1986.

Shizuto Masunaga with Waturu Ohasi, *Zen Shiatsu*, Japan Publications Inc, Tokyo Japan, 1983.

Miyamoto Musashi, *A Book of Five Rings*, Allison and Busby, 1983.

Toru Namikoshi, *The Complete Book of Shiatsu Therapy*, Japan Publications Inc, Tokyo Japan, 1984.

FACIAL DIAGNOSIS

There is growing interest in this method of diagnosis which originates from Eastern healthcare philosophies and forms an important part of traditional Chinese medicine.

Careful observation of the face and tongue can point towards the condition of the whole body in much the same way as iridologists and reflexologists look to the eyes and to the feet. It is particularly useful in that it requires no tools or techniques, and with the aid of just a mirror can become a useful way of assessing one's own state of health.

We use facial diagnosis all the time, in a small way, whenever we look at another and recognise that they're looking pale or have been crying or have good colour in their cheeks. This has simply been developed and a map of the body imposed upon the colour judgements which we make naturally. It makes such good sense to 'read' this wholly accessible part of the body and so make a preliminary diagnosis, or confirm findings; it's easy and straightforward, and the patient need not undress or be subjected to any form of manipulation or investigation.

The skin colour, condition and texture are all taken into consideration, alongside an assessment of the features and any particular markings. The face is divided into areas relating to the internal organs and body systems. Their state can then be assessed according to the type of marking or degree of colour present in each area. One clear example of this is the area under the eyes which is said to relate to the kidneys. This is a site which can become puffy when we are retaining water and which shows when we have been drinking more than a usual amount of alcohol in the slightly darker than usual bags or rings.

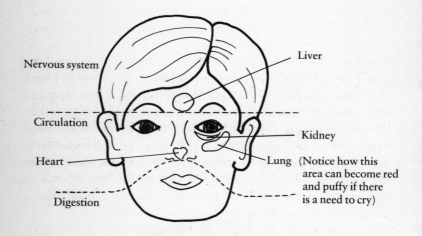

General areas and markings for facial diagnosis

Different races obviously have different basic skin colours, but the colour characteristics of any imbalance remain the same, although practice is needed to discern them. The presence of white spots, for example, can point to an over-consumption of dairy products, whereas a general greyish colouring can indicate an under-active liver. This is most common in Western, industrialised countries where the liver is under enormous additional pressure from environmental pollutants and high levels of food additives.

Skin texture may be assessed as rough, oily, dry, wet, etc.

Rough skin can result from an excess of saturated fats in the diet, which makes extra work for the liver and kidneys. Dry skin may be caused by higher than usual cholesterol levels or, conversely, by a lack of oil and fat soluble vitamins.

As a general rule, sore, dry or red skin indicates a condition of internal heat, whereas clammy or moist skin usually points to a colder constitution. These factors are important in terms of diagnosing and treating any illnesses that the patient may manifest. They conform to the Chinese system of analysing most situations as either yin (cold) or yang (hot). This is similar to the diagnosis Shiatsu practitioners make of kyo (empty) or jitsu (full). These terms can apply to all areas of life, where the yang principle would be experienced as contracting, light-giving, masculine etc., and the yin principle as expansive, dark, feminine etc. All things may be seen as having a pre-dominance of yin or yang, and the balance between these opposites is perhaps best illustrated by the well-known symbol which incorporates both within the wholeness of the circle.

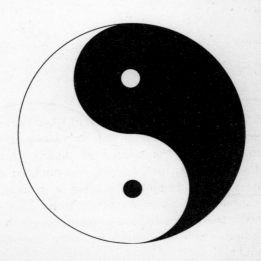

Yin and Yang illustration

Once this condition is ascertained, the appropriate dietary, exercise and lifestyle changes can be introduced. Yin people tend to feel cold, for example, and will respond well to warming spices added to the diet, whereas these should be avoided for a yang individual.

The size, shape, positioning and symmetry of the features are also of great importance. Eyebrows, for instance, can be classified as close together, far apart, upward or downward slanting, peaked, etc., all reflecting different constitutional types. Overall, they are said to show the condition of the nervous, digestive, respiratory, circulatory and excretory systems, so they can reveal constitutional states developed during gestation as well as current conditions. The left brow is said to reflect the paternal and the right brow the maternal influences, and they are further divided to indicate stages of development. The thickness of eyebrow hair shows the degree of basic vitality and can also demonstrate strength of character (an interesting implication for those who pluck their brows!).

Left
Paternal influences

Right
Maternal influences

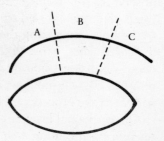

A = Early development, either foetal or youth
B = Mid-part of development, either foetal or middle age
C = Late part of development, either foetal or old age

The lips relate to the digestive system and the sexual organs (consider a moustache!). The lower lip serves as an indicator for the intestines, the upper lip for the stomach and genitals. A slightly swollen lower lip may indicate constipation and crust formation in the corners of the mouth may result through difficulties with fat metabolism.

The tongue is a good indicator of overall health and this can be easily seen if you look at your own tongue every morning; comparing its colour and degree of coating through good health, periods of ill health and 'mornings after'. This can prove very revealing; confirming how well the body is working. The coating is generally a sign that the body is detoxifying or cleansing itself, and liver function (the main organ of detoxification) can be observed along the sides of the tongue.

In keeping with its Chinese origins, some facial signs are reputed to indicate the energetic state of the organ or body part to which they relate. This can then point to imbalances or difficulties before they manifest physically. To this end, many emotional states and vitality observations can be made by an experienced practitioner.

It is well worth taking another look at people's faces; observing, for instance, the size and positioning of the ears (high placement is said to indicate intelligence), and the depth of the lines connecting the nose to the corners of the mouth — the career lines. More practitioners are now using this form of diagnosis as an aid in determining the condition and the progress of their patients, and as a useful way of involving the patient in the process of their own healthcare.

On a personal level, it can be used to provide an immediate reference — pointing to periods of excess or under-nourishment, and as an aid to understanding how to maintain energy levels. Although professional assistance is needed to diagnose constitutional states and any disease process accurately, a thorough look at your face using this method can prove beneficial on an everyday level.

Yang foods, such as cooked grains, pulses, sea vegetables and fish can be added to the diet if extra concentration or concerted effort is required for a short period of time. Yin foods – leafy green vegetables, fruits and salads generally – can then help you wind down afterwards. It is well worth experimenting with these simple dietary measures.

Finding out more

Community Health Foundation
188 Old Street
London EC1V 9BP
Tel: 071 251 4076

Further reading

Oliver and Michele Cowmeadow, *Yin Yang Cookbook*, Optima, 1988.

Michio Kushi, *Your Face Never Lies*, Avery, 1990.

FLOWER REMEDIES

The distilled essences of flowers can be used for their therapeutic effects on both the emotional and physical levels.

A retired English doctor, Edward Bach, first started to use these flower essences or remedies at the turn of this century. He combined his knowledge of psychological typing and emotional states with his love of nature and began to explore the therapeutic use of flowers. On his early morning walks, he collected the dew which had settled on the petals of an assortment of flowers and explored their effects on his own emotions. Through time he evolved a system of determining the effects of a number of different flowers and set about making the remedies available commercially.

He experimented with letting the petals steep in water and then exposing them to sunlight to allow the preparation to be infused with the healing qualities of the flowers. He later added alcohol as a preservative so that they could be bottled and, now, exported around the world.

His theory that different diseases were directly related to emotional types or temperaments led him to make seven classifications of personality, which are then sub-divided to make a specific diagnosis easier. His definitions were over-sensitivity, fear, uncertainty or indecision, lack of interest in the present, despondency and despair, over-concern for the welfare of others, and loneliness.

Over sensitivity, for example, has four different remedies – agrimony for anxiety and mental torment hidden by a brave face; centaury for a weak will or co-dependent habits; walnut for major life changes and holly for jealousy and suspicion.

Perhaps his most well-known combination of flower essences is 'Rescue Remedy' – a mixture of five different remedies: cherry plum, clematis, impatiens, rock rose and Star of Bethlehem. This was designed as the perfect first-aid measure for shock and anxiety. To quote Bach's own writings, 'It is an all-purpose composite for effects of anguish, examinations, going to the dentist, etc. Comforting, calming and reassuring to those distressed by startling experiences.' Its use, though, is restricted to non-medical emergencies because of the alcohol content of the mixture, although it can be used externally in such instances and has been proven to be extremely effective when used in this way.

Since this pioneering work, the use of flower essences has been developed further, incorporating flowers from different parts of the world. The many varieties now available are known as Flower Essences, marking them as distinct from the Bach Flower Remedies.

The small 10 or 20ml bottles in which the remedies or essences are sold each contain a dropper and the idea is to take two or three drops on the tongue, or in a small glass of water which is then very slowly sipped. With some remedies, particularly Rescue Remedy, the effect can be felt immediately, although they all have a long-term effect too.

Those working on depression, chronic situations or deep-seated feelings can all be taken regularly – first thing in the morning, last thing at night and two or three times during the day – to achieve the best results. Many of the remedies can also be taken for the fleeting moods of everyday life. The simplest way to do this is to mix a little of the remedy or remedies of your choice with some spring water and keep them in a small dropper bottle – these can be bought at any pharmacy.

The remedies can be used externally too – a few drops of elm added to hot water in which a compress is soaked can provide tremendous ease for strained or pulled ligaments when applied to the area. Crab apple can be added to a cold water wash for boils or bad spots, and Rescue Remedy applied to a bruise speeds up resolution. Its use in this way became so popular that there is now available a lanolin-free cream. Rescue Remedy, either in cream or the liquid form is also an excellent first-aid remedy for minor burns; a few drops on the burn itself and one on the tongue soon promote total recovery.

The remedies can be used by children – again bearing in mind the alcohol content – as an excellent first-aid remedy for the trauma of minor accidents. They are also said to be quite effective for treating animals and also plants. A few drops of rescue remedy added to the water for a distressed plant should soon pep it up.

A list of the full range of flower remedies can be obtained wherever the remedies are sold, and each essence is itemised alongside a few key words to enable self-diagnosis. Many counsellors and therapists use flower remedies alongside their work. These can help ease or resolve painful feelings as they come up.

The remedies can be taken at any time and there are no contra-indications to their use, except that they contain alcohol, which may prohibit their use by some people. Because you only take a small amount at a time – usually just a few drops – the alcohol content should not stop you driving or fulfilling any other tasks.

Dr Bach also worked as a homoeopath and as such was used to dealing with the subtler aspects of medicine. He was content to state that the healing energy of the flowers transferred itself to the water solution in which they were soaked. Having a small bottle of the remedy was, obviously, easier than having to find the flower itself, particularly for those not living in the countryside or without the knowledge to identify each plant correctly. The bottling of remedies also meant that each remedy would be available throughout the year, not just when the flower itself was in bloom.

Today we eat the flowers, leaves, stems and roots of plants for their nutritious and health-giving qualities, and bathe in the fragrance of their essential oils, so it is only a small step to accepting that the water in which flower petals sit in the preparation of each remedy can easily absorb their potent qualities.

I keep some remedies close to hand – my own favourites are: Rescue Remedy for trauma; crab apple for its cleansing qualities; rock rose for fear and terror (terrific for stage fright!); and olive for fatigue. People soon find their own favourites, and those which help at different times.

Flower Remedies and essences are available at many health food shops, chemists and natural health clinics.

Finding out more

The Edward Bach Centre
Mount Vernon
Sotwell
Wallingford
Oxon OX10 0PZ
Tel: 0491 39489 / 34678

Flower Essence Society
PO Box 459
Nevada City
California 95959
USA
Tel: (800) 548 0075 or (916) 265 0258

Further reading

Edward Bach, *Heal Thyself*, C.W. Daniel Company, 1946.

Julian Barnard, *A Guide to the Bach Flower Remedies*, C.W. Daniel Company, 1979.

Julian Barnard, *Patterns of Life Force: A Review of the Life and Work of Dr Edward Bach*, Bach Educational Programme, Hereford, 1987.

GROUP WORK

There must be nearly as many reasons for joining a group as there are different groups to join! In the main, these can be divided into three broad categories: to learn a particular skill or set of skills, e.g. assertiveness training; to seek to resolve a particular situation that involves others, e.g. family therapy; to share experiences and a support network, e.g. growth groups. Being in a group can, in part, satisfy our basic human need for contact and social interaction.

The structure and regularity of meetings will vary – sometimes a leader, facilitator or trainer will provide a focus for the group, or the organisation and input will be shared by all. Most often a commitment is required as far as attendance is concerned, although some groups are far more informal, operating on an 'as needed' or drop-in basis. This is most often the case with support organisations such as Alcoholics Anonymous and Narcotics Anonymous.

The women's consciousness-raising groups I worked with in the 1970s used a completely open structure – with people committing to one meeting at a time, no chairperson and the venue alternating among the homes of the members. This apparent lack of formal structure encouraged the personal responsibility and individual contribution of all involved.

Obviously the structure and agenda of any group will to a large degree be determined by its cause – why the group has formed – but there are many common factors. In groups we may learn more about the way we relate to others, how those interactions affect us, and how we are perceived by others. The inevitable exchange of views, opinions and feelings can lead to improved social skills and a greater self-knowledge, whether or not these are direct aims.

The support and understanding offered by many groups can build confidence and create a secure forum in which to express one's deeper feelings. If membership is mixed in terms of age, gender, interests, social background, etc., then the group can become a microcosm of society, proving to be a sample of reality in which new stances and forms of expression can be explored. More defined groups – those with a particular purpose or specific membership – can provide a unique opportunity for solidarity.

The prospect of joining a group can be daunting for some, conjuring up embarrassing memories of school-time pressures to 'contribute'. The warm, supportive nature of most groups, however, soon puts people at their ease. Most often there is no pressure to speak or participate actively, although some groups begin by going round and giving everybody the opportunity to introduce themselves, often just by saying their name.

Of course not all groups are growth-related – nor do they need to be to provide the benefits of working closely with others. With the purpose of making social contacts and interacting with others, a host of activity-based groups is available – from formalized rôle-playing as in amateur dramatic societies, to re-enactment situations like the Tolkien society (they gather and act out situations from his books; often meeting over weekends and setting up living and social conditions to fit each theme). These could be seen as the ultimate in play therapy!

Gatherings of any people who share a common interest, whether it be archery, a health condition, or a life purpose, provide a valuable opportunity to understand more about ourselves and how we function in society. As a rule, most people gain from joining with others in this way in direct proportion to their openness to new ideas and the generosity with which they share their own experiences.

To name just a few, there are encounter groups, therapy groups, family groups, those that meet to discuss dream analysis, to meditate, to learn the physical expression of their feelings, and for mutual support. Information about local and national groups can be found in libraries, Citizens Advice Bureaux and adult education centres.

Common to all growth-related groups is the sense of making a safe and confidential place where support or whatever is needed can be received. It can be very reassuring to hear one's own fears or anxieties being voiced by other people; and this can help us all gain some perspective on our own discomfort. For those without any particular worries, groups can often provide the opportunity to refine our skills in establishing relationships.

In groups with a specific purpose, assertiveness training for example, all other group members will be involved in acting out potential situations and practising their responses. This can lead to real breakthroughs in that the insights and actions of a wide range of people can be focused to provide some truly effective strategies.

Family therapy and other problem-solving endeavours benefit from the objectivity of the group facilitator or therapist. To change familiar patterns of behaviour requires us first to notice them – something we often need either distance or the observations of an onlooker to achieve. The old cliché of not seeing the wood for the trees is most pertinent when applied to relationship situations. Although most effective when all involved parties are present within the group, much headway can be made with only some family members being present, or even with only one partner in the case of a partnership.

Loneliness is a growing problem in our society. The more

complex, industrialised and urban our living conditions, the more isolation people are inclined to feel. With the breakdown of local communities and ever smaller family units our need for company becomes greater. The real gift of group situations is in the opportunity they provide for people to truly meet, to share what is important to them as individuals whilst leaving behind a lot of the labels, to step out of any constraining rôles they must play in their everyday lives and be themselves.

Finding out more

Institute of Family Therapy
43 New Cavendish Street
London W1
Tel: 071 935 1651.

Overeaters Anonymous
c/o Manor Gardens Centre
609, Manor Gardens
London N7
Tel: 081 868 4109

Alcoholics Anonymous
11 Radcliffe Gardens
London SW10
Tel: 081 352 3001

Institute for Dream Analysis
1 Daleham Gardens
Hampstead
London NW3 5BY
Tel: 071 431 2693

WILL (Worshop Institute for Living Learning)
218 Randolph Avenue
London W9
Tel: 071 328 8955

HEALING

Healing is, in a sense, what all of this book is concerned with: not really to do with fixing or repairing, but about uniting mind, body and spirit in a balanced, health-giving way.

There are many forms of natural healing exchange; it can take place between a mother and child, between lovers, or friends who care deeply for each other. This is a natural, human thing, and it occurs spontaneously when needed. Healing is also a personal process; we heal ourselves constantly from birth. We may, however, seek help from others on occasions, or encounter it, but any personal transformation is by its very nature an individual thing.

Healers help others by providing the energy that is needed for the patient or client to heal themselves. This may take the form of physical work, or emotional support, or counselling; the important thing is that it is backed by genuine care, and can be easily received. As self-righting organisms we take what we need in order to facilitate our own healing.

Some healers call themselves faith healers or spiritualist healers. For some faith healers, that they believe it works is enough; others require the person receiving the healing to have faith in them. There is an important distinction between spiritual healers, who maintain that their work is spiritually inspired, and Spiritualist healers who believe that they are used by healing spirits and have their own church and organised religious beliefs.

Many healers simply call themselves healers or psychic or natural healers. All healing is natural. Most psychics who work as healers place an emphasis on the counselling aspect of any work they do, believing that conscious awareness of the nature of any difficulty – how it arose, what compounds it, etc., is an integral part of any healing process. There is no point in repairing something if you don't know how it got upset in the first place. Without such knowledge, there is every possibility of it occurring again.

Although many of the lessons that we need to learn in life may have to be repeated, we can avoid a lot of unnecessary time and energy expenditure by completing things properly. This often means reaching back to find the cause of any complaint, and psychics can also help by discovering the level of any disorder – its root may be inherited, physical and affected by diet, for example, or it may be emotional, or energetic. Some of our problems can be caused, or at least compounded, by a lack of understanding. This again is where the counselling can help by bringing other matters to our attention.

Healing sessions will vary according to the type of healer. Often they involve 'hands-on' work, when the healer will gently touch the body at a variety of sites, others hold their hands near the body.

Many healers include other techniques – they may have studied some form of healthcare, perhaps physically-based like cranio-sacral therapy, or maybe more system-related like herbalism or naturopathy. They can then combine their knowledge with their healing ability to work using any number of techniques.

When using hands-on work, the healer may use both their hands to 'sandwich' particular parts of the body, or they may be placed some distance apart. People describe the feelings as being warming, or tingling; some find a refreshing coolness under the healer's hands, and memories or thoughts may come into the mind. Sometimes people see images or colours weaving themselves around the healer and themselves. Each experience is different – those needing to find peace usually feel calm and restful, a depressed individual may feel pleasantly energised after a session. Some people may not be aware of any sensations at all, but feel somewhat different or changed afterwards.

This work can also be done without touching the patient or client. Healers work mainly by interacting with a person's energy and this extends beyond the body to form the aura. Some psychics can see this, others feel it or sense it, and many find they prefer to work in this way. Once again, the person receiving the healing may be aware of changes in temperature or a variety of sensations, including emotional releases during the session. Usually these take place with the client seated, but they can be lying down on a treatment couch, or even standing.

A person's energy can be seen by some psychics to emanate from a number of centres. The major ones, sometimes called chakras, are in a midline extending from above the head down through the whole body. Each centre relates to a different drive or motivational energy, e.g. courage, creativity, inspiration, etc. These centres, being comprised of energy, also have a colour, a sound or harmonic, a texture, etc. Many psychics see or sense the colours and use this information to assess a person's overall health. A grass green relates to the creativity centre; yellow relates to the solar or courage centre; pink to emotional and physical energy from the heart centre; mauve to the communication centre; blue to the centre for motivation or inspiration.

Quartz crystals can help encourage, support and rebalance the energy centres; rose quartz is good for the heart centre which houses emotion, and sapphire for the inspiration centre which is located in the head. Quartz crystals are sometimes used during a session or you may see one on the healer's desk. Quartz crystal works as a battery, and the energy from the healer can connect with the energy of the quartz and transfer it to the client. Psychics may also wear a crystal or gemstone, and they can use the quartz as a pendulum to aid diagnosis.

Some healers used coloured lights to impress the consciousness of the client, some use little black boxes and do not necessarily call themselves healers.

Healing energy can also be transmitted over long distances – the receiver can be miles away or in another country. Many healers keep absent or distant healing lists, and they will send healing energy to people who are experiencing difficulties but cannot see the healer in person.

Some people believe that the ability to heal is a gift and as such it must be freely given. These people either work for nothing or accept donations. Many healers realise that we have to give and receive (there is balance in this action, as in all others) and, like all other practitioners, charge or take donations for their sessions. These usually last between thirty minutes and one hour, although timings do vary.

There are no associations that cover the whole profession, mainly because of the wide range of different techniques that healers use. Individual knowledge, interpretation skills and beliefs vary as enormously in this profession as does expertise. It is important to find a healer with whom you feel at ease. Personal referral is generally the way to find a healer, or you could approach the Spiritualist church.

Further reading

Betty Balcombe, *As I See it*, Balcombe Books, 1986

Gerald Jampoulski, *Love is Letting Go of Fear*, Foundation for Inner Peace, 1986

W. Brugh Joy, *Joy's Way*, J.P. Tarcher Inc, 1982.

Bernie Siegel, *Love, Medicine and Miracles*, Harper & Row, 1980.

HERBS

The use of herbs and plants for their nutritional and curative properties is a well-documented part of our history. Herbs were our earliest form of medicine. Their nutritional benefits and healing powers have been known for centuries. From the papyrus documents of ancient Egypt and the earliest Chinese writings come detailed records of the uses and values of a variety of plants and herbs, many of which are still used today. Many of the herbs now commonly used in Europe travelled from the Mediterranean courtesy of the Egyptians and the Romans, but each continent has its own indigenous plants.

Nowadays, our laboratories are busy distilling the active properties of plants for use in the pharmaceutical industry. Much of the medication currently available is copied or extracted from nature: digitalis, a powerful heart drug, from foxgloves; quinine from the bark of the cinchona tree; cancer-inhibiting drugs from tropical plants; pain-killers from poppies and aspirin from the willow tree. Some 25 per cent of modern medicines are synthetic copies of the active constituents of plants. As medical science investigates further, so new discoveries are made and then copied or synthesised, concentrated and provided to the public, in a form that bears little resemblance to the original natural remedy.

Many naturopaths use herbs extensively and there is a host of herbs that can be used in the home. In the main, these will be eaten fresh or dried, and can be added to meals or drunk as infusions or teas. They can also be applied externally as compresses or poultices, or diluted to form valuable washes and added to baths.

Many modern herbalists or medical herbalists tend to work exclusively with herbs, although some will also use wider dietary measures. They will most usually prescribe the herbs as tinctures or decoctions (liquids that are distillations of the herbs themselves mixed with alcohol). This means that they can be taken as a 'medicine' – one 5 ml dose twice a day, for example – although this method makes it difficult for those with any alcohol intolerance.

The old school herbalist, however, will often have a much wider appreciation of the use and preparation of herbs and their role in the diet. They are more likely to suggest other health-promoting measures and have a keen knowledge of the need for proper diet, elimination and exercise to enhance the work of the herbs themselves. This is where you are likely to encounter a richness of remedies and a much wider variety of medicinal forms, including elixirs, cordials, boluses, syrups and tisanes.

Practitioners of Chinese herbal medicine use Oriental herbs alongside wider dietary measures. They diagnose according to traditional Chinese principles, assessing the nature of the individual, the disorder and the chosen herbs and diet in terms of their energetic value – hot or cold, yin or yang (see page 89).

Herbs have a toning effect on the tissues of the body and are often able to restore function to disordered or imbalanced organs and systems. Individual herbs will have an affinity with a particular organ or system: parsley is a kidney tonic; dandelion a liver tonic; and red clover has a cleansing action on the lymphatic system. Some of the herbs' efficacy can be attributed to their vitamin and mineral content, which will be easily taken up by the body. Nettles are particularly high in iron, and rosehips are a good source of vitamin C.

Each herb or plant comprises a sometimes complicated group of properties, and this balance of active and inactive ingredients can aid absorption and prevent against side-effects. (The majority of herbs have none, the few that do will be handled with care by a trained practitioner.) Side-effects do occur, however, when the active constituents are isolated or concentrated, as in pharmaceutical drugs. Herbs have a rapid action in the body and it is important to combine them correctly and monitor their amount or dosage and frequency in order to gain their full benefit. Over-dosage is rarely dangerous, again unlike the synthetic versions.

Psychics and some other people can have a high level of sensitivity or affinity with herbs as well as with other forms of medicine and treatment. By eating or taking herbs in their natural form, it is easy to control the amount and frequency of intake, and therefore the beneficial effects. As a general rule, the fresh herb will be most active and effective, although careful drying preserves many of the herbs' properties and is the most suitable method for storage. Once dried, the herbs need to be protected from light and heat if they are not to deteriorate.

The use of herbs can be short-term and specific or more general and on-going. Fresh or dried yarrow may be taken as a tea several times a day to help with a case of cystitis, yet it may also be recommended as an ongoing support – a cup once or twice a week throughout the season to continue cleansing the area.

Although most herbs can be taken internally in this way, a number can be very effective when applied externally.

Calendula or marigold is an excellent skin healer and its cleansing action makes it suitable for use anywhere on the body. I often recommend its addition to the bath in cases of vaginal infection:

Take 4 oz of dried calendula and add to a gallon of water. Allow to sit for twelve hours and bring to a gentle boil. Simmer for six minutes then strain the liquid into a hot bath and discard the flower heads. Sit in the bath, ensuring the kidney area is immersed, for about twenty minutes, then wrap up and go straight to bed.

A macerated cabbage leaf is another tremendous skin cleanser – its leeching effect makes it a useful poultice for boils or deep spots:

Place a cabbage leaf in boiling water for thirty seconds (larger, more sinewy leaves may need up to forty-five seconds). Place the leaf directly onto the spot, as hot as it tolerable, or if the skin is broken apply between two pieces of thin gauze. Cover with a warm bandage or towel and leave in place for up to two hours. This can be repeated as necessary.

A very old-fashioned remedy is to crush some fresh comfrey leaves and place as a compress or add to the splint for a broken bone. The comfrey or bone-knit would also be taken internally with a meal or as a tea to facilitate healing.

The table overleaf shows the home applications of some common herbs, many of which you may be used to adding to meals for their culinary properties. Herbs used in cooking often have a particular effect on digestion – the caraway, cardamom and other seeds found in curried sauces prevent flatulence. The cloves that are so regularly added to winter meals are excellent

for the circulation and nutmeg sprinkled on night-time drinks
is a natural tranquilliser.

All of these herbs are safe to use as first-aid measures,
although this form of prescription should never be substituted
for a visit to a practitioner. If the measure is not effective, or
the condition recurs, this could be a symptom of another
complaint, so use these herbs with discretion.

Care must always be taken during pregnancy and herbs
should not be taken without the advice and monitoring of a
healthcare practitioner.

Herb	Properties	Home uses
Calendula or Marigold	Extensive healing properties, particularly for skin and in the treatment of fungal conditions	As a cream for cuts and grazes. Added to the bath or as a gargle for thrush. As a tea: taken weekly for internal cleansing and healing
Chamomile	Calming, eliminating, digestive	Soothing for the nervous system. As a tea can help relieve billiousness and flatulence. A good after-dinner drink. The cold tea makes a soothing eye wash
Fennel	Soothing for digestion and sore throats	A main constituent of gripe water, can be taken as a weak tea to aid digestion. Good as a gargle

Lady's mantle	A 'women's' herb	As a tea: brings energy to the pelvis, helps regulate periods and strengthen the womb. Can also be added to bath water (as directions in text for calendula)
Marjoram	Sedative, relaxing	As a tea: good for period pain, nervous headache and acid digestion. Not more than one cup a day. To relieve pain of colic: heat the dried herb and wrap around the abdomen in a tea towel or similar
Nettle	High in iron. Blood purifier, stimulates production of fresh blood cells	Good for all skin complaints resulting from toxins or sluggish elimination. As a tea, good during menstruation and to help prevent anaemia.
Parsley	Cleansing, high in iron	Add to meals
Peppermint	Digestive, stimulating	Warming in winter, a good after-dinner drink. Useful if bowel movements are sluggish

Red sage	Excellent for throats	As a gargle for sore throats and a mouth-wash for ulcers and sore gums. As a tea for upper bronchial complaints
Rosemary	Antiseptic, cleansing	Use in cooking and as an inhalant for breathing difficulties (particularly sinus conditions). As a tea: a good headache cure, and will help relieve muscle cramping and spasm. Useful as an anti-fungal treatment
Slippery Elm	A powerful, soothing emulcant	Made into a paste with a little water or apple juice has a soothing effect on digestion. Useful for tummy upsets, or irritated bowel
St John's Wort	Excellent for skin and external use	Soak the leaves in oil then brush it on to varicose veins, bruises and rough skin to speed healing
Yarrow	Promotes sweating, aids kidney function, promotes production of fresh blood cells in the bone marrow	In Sitz bath to aid elimination through the kidneys. As a tea for cystitis and to relieve diarrhoea.

Finding out more

British Herbal Medicine Association
Lane House
Cowling
Keighley
West Yorkshire BD22 0LX

Dr Christopher School of Natural Healing
19 Park Terrace
Stoke on Trent
Staffordshire

National Institute of Medical Herbalists
41 Hatherley Road
Winchester
Hampshire SO22 6RR
Tel: 0962 68776

Further reading

Kitty Campion, *Kitty Campion's Handbook of Herbal Health*, Sphere Books, 1985.

Nicholas Culpepper, *Culpepper's Complete Herbal*, W. Foulsham and Co Ltd.

Barbara Griggs, *The Home Herbal*, Pan Books, 1982.

David Hoffman, *The Holistic Herbal*, Element, 1983.

Richard Mabey (cons. ed.), *The Complete New Herbal*, Gaia/Elm Tree, 1988.

Anne McIntyre, *Herbal Medicine*, Optima, 1987.

Maria Treben, *Health from God's Garden*, Thorsons, 1987.

HYDROTHERAPY

**Drinking water · Inhalations · Showers · Douches
Enemas · Sitz baths**

This is the use of water as a therapeutic agent. Used internally, but most often externally, water can be applied hot, warm or cold; under pressure, for partial immersion or local use. This natural therapy has been used for centuries, and its immediate effectiveness and ease of application make it a valuable tool for home healthcare.

It is important to provide our bodies with sufficient water each day, and drinking fresh, clean water is the fastest, most effective way to do this. Unfortunately, this description does not fit the tap water available in many countries, including Britain, so it needs to be filtered, or passed over in favour of bottled mineral waters.

Water has a myriad of external uses too – making use of its thermal qualities, cold packs and compresses have an immediate first-aid application for injuries. Applying a cotton cloth (tea-towel or handkerchief) that has been soaked in cold water to a muscle spasm or bruise has instant beneficial effects. The cold encourages the body to rush fresh blood supplies to the area; this brings additional oxygen and nutrients to the site so that the body can then begin its process of repair.

Steam inhalations, an old-fashioned remedy, are often used to relieve chest congestion, but these are particularly beneficial for any skin complaints as well as providing help and relief for sore throats and mucus conditions. You can buy facial saunas at any electrical shop, but these are not necessary to benefit fully from this treatment. You can do it yourself quite easily with a kettle, a bowl and a towel.

Add boiling water to a large bowl and bend your head over it, covering your head and the bowl with a large towel to stop the steam from escaping. Breathe in through your nose as well as through your mouth, and try to stay under the towel for as long as possible. If you get too hot, then lift your head out from time to time for a breath of cooler air, but leave the bowl covered so that none of the steam is lost.

There are various botanicals you can add to the water, but the steam alone is remarkably effective at clearing sinuses and relieving tight chests. Rosemary is particularly antiseptic, and a stem of the fresh herb rubbed between the fingers (to release its aromatic oil) and then added to the water will bring speedy relief to chesty coughs and will also loosen congestion in the sinuses. One drop of the essential oil of rosemary could be used instead, or one drop of Olbas oil. Rosemary is also a great astringent, so those with oily skin or pimples will benefit from this inhalation, which can be repeated daily.

Red sage is another herb which lends itself to being used in this way. It will cleanse and tone the mucous membranes and is particularly useful for soothing sore throats. This is a relative of common sage, most often used for its culinary benefits.

White thyme and tea tree oil are more forceful in their action, and one drop of either of these essential oils added to the inhalation will be an excellent first-aid measure against any virus conditions. The oils of eucalyptus and peppermint are effective at clearing stuffy noses and shifting a dry cough. A few rose petals or a drop of essential oil of rose make a soothing inhalation which is particularly good for softening a wind- or sun-dried skin.

Regular plain steam inhalations can form an important part of the treatment of any bronchial complaint and can be useful in the treatment of asthma. It if is not possible to perform the procedure as advised, then the steam from an open kettle or from a running hot water tap can still be of assistance. In a small room, with the doors and windows closed, this steam will be inhaled and can help make breathing easier. A person with any breathing difficulty may well be feeling anxious and shutting them in like this should not be attempted if there are any feelings of claustrophobia or insecurity.

The use of **showers** or shower sprays is a valuable addition to the treatment of any part of the body. By varying the temperature of the water, your body will be encouraged to speed up its overall circulation, and fresh nutrients will be brought quickly to the area being sprayed. This is particularly effective in speeding up the resolution of bruises and hastens the recovery time of any sprains or strains. It can also relieve pelvic congestion when used on the abdominal area, or act as a general circulation enhancer if used all over on a regular basis.

The golden rule when varying the temperature of the water is always to finish with cold; so when spraying, start with warm water, then switch to cold for one minute, then back to warm, then cold again for another minute. This can be repeated up to five times, making sure to end with a cold spray, and the whole process can be repeated up to three times each day.

If a shower head is not available, the same effect can be achieved with two bowls of water, one hot and one cold or even directly under the taps if the body part to be treated is small.

Another wonderfully invigorating use of shower sprays is as

something strangely called a Scottish douche. A high-pressure shower head is aimed along the length of the spine, using first hot water, then cold. This directly stimulates the nerves as they leave the bony protection of the spine and move to supply the rest of the body. The easiest way to achieve this is with someone's assistance, although with careful positioning of the shower head and by moving yourself up and down, it can be done on your own. The dramatic effects are felt straight away and it is advisable to allow a few minutes rest immediately afterwards, and not to do this more than once a day, unless resting.

Vaginal **douches** have encountered some bad press in recent years, but this is mainly as a result of their incorrect use. The only safe douche is a gravity one – this uses the pull of gravity to govern the flow of liquid and its exit from the body. The absence of any pressure or force ensures that no damage is done to the delicate vaginal walls and that the cervix will remain untroubled.

The douche comprises a bag or rigid container which is filled with water, or water mixed with other substances, and hung on a shower rail or wall hook; a longish tube that runs from it, and a small, removable nozzle with small perforations at its end. While standing or crouching in the bath, the nozzle is inserted into the vagina and a slow, steady flow flushes the water through and out of the body. Douches are obtainable from any chemist.

A douche solution made of nine parts warm water to one part apple cider vinegar can be remarkably helpful in the treatment of vaginal thrush. The use of tepid water can help improve the tone of vaginal muscles after pregnancy or dramatic weight loss. Care must be taken at all times, and particularly after pregnancy, when you should not douche without first checking with a healthcare practitioner.

Douching is hopelessly ineffective as a means of contraception, often having the reverse effect and making conception more likely. It can, though, be a useful adjunct to overall healthcare, and some women find it especially useful in restoring their body's delicate balance after the use of contraceptive creams and gells.

Enemas work in essentially the same way, and most douche kits will include a separate nozzle for insertion into the anus. When using enemas, the same amount of care is needed as for douching, so as not to damage the delicate lining of this sensitive area. Enemas are most often taken whilst lying down, and in the past, played an important role in many medical practices. Doctors and health practitioners would recommend them, and the practice nurse would carry out the procedure in the surgery. Nowadays they are most often used at home.

Their effect on clearing the bowel is dramatic and for this reason their use is not recommended on too regular a basis. Two or three enemas should clear any particular obstructive problem, but they should not be substituted for proper dietary care. If used too frequently (more than once a month), the body can come to rely upon them, rather than using them for assistance in times of need. The enema is quite safe if gravity assisted – this means there is no pressure used and the flow of water is governed by the rate at which it passes naturally down the pipe and into the body. Colonic irrigation is currently growing in popularity – this is something quite different to an enema. Here water is pumped high into the colon under pressure, and is often aerated or has other substances added to it. I cannot stress enough the need to have one's condition properly diagnosed before considering this procedure, and that it must be performed by a qualified practitioner. That they have trained on the equipment used is not sufficient qualification to allow a person to treat such a delicate and important area of the body in this way. They must also have the anatomical and physiological knowledge necessary for correct diagnosis.

In more general use, water as therapy has many applications. A hot bath at the end of a long day warms and relaxes the body, and provides a useful transition time before sleeping. Cold water run over the wrists on a hot day cools and calms the whole body, and an early morning paddle in cold water stimulates and wakes up the body remarkably well.

The **sitz bath** is a wonderful way of invigorating the whole body; improving the circulation and the immune system and relieving the nervous system. It is particularly useful in conditions of pelvic congestion or if there are any spinal lesions in the low back. A bowl large enough to sit in is needed – a baby bath is ideal. This is filled with cold water and placed in a bath filled with about one foot of hot water. The idea is to sit in one temperature, say the cold water, making sure that the water covers the hips up to the waist completely, with the feet immersed in another temperature – the hot water. After one or two minutes change places, so that the pelvis is now in hot water and the feet in cold. Make at least one more change over and finish with the pelvis in cold water, the feet in hot. Whilst bathing, make sure the whole pelvic area is covered by splashing water up over the abdomen and between the legs. Finish off with a brisk towel rub and allow a short time to relax after this dynamic treatment.

Finding out more

British Naturopathic Association
6 Netherhall Gardens
London NW3 5RR
Tel: 071 435 6464

Incorporated Society of British Naturopaths
Kingston
The Couch House
293 Gilmerton Road
Edinburgh EH16 5UQ
Tel: 031 664 3435

Further reading

Henry Lindlahr, *Natural Therapeutics Volume II Practice*,
C.W. Daniel Company, 1975.

IONS

The air around us is full of neutral, positively and negatively charged particles called ions. It is the negative ions which are the most beneficial; an over-abundance of positive ions contributing to a number of health concerns, mood changes and energy slumps.

The ion concentration present in the air we breathe is determined by a number of factors. Many natural elements increase the number of negative ions in the surrounding air – fire and water being two of the most effective. This partly explains the restful, invigorating nature of an evening spent in front of a real fire, and the feelings of expansion and renewal when close to a waterfall or any body of moving water. Actually, any natural environment is likely to have a more beneficial ionisation than a synthetic one. Mountains have cleaner air than offices, on this we can all agree, but recognising that the ion concentration is a major factor in this state of affairs allows us to begin to redress that imbalance.

The synthetic fabric in curtains, carpets and furnishings; dust, cigarette smoke and other airborne particles; TV sets and VDU screens all increase the number of positively charged ions in the atmosphere. That means that all city air has high positive ion concentrations and that just about all homes and places of work do too.

The effects of this are important in relation to healthcare. Large amounts of negative ions have a lethal effect on bacteria, making for a cleaner environment. They effect the levels of various neuro-hormones in the blood and they reduce the level of histamine, giving relief to people with nervous tension and allergic responses. They also seem to affect the normal human circadian rhythm – the rise and fall of both physical and psychological energy throughout the day. Studies have shown that the energy dips previously considered as normal disappear in a highly negatively ionised environment.

The changes in mood and minor health complaints that people experience when there are sudden weather changes has led to detailed study into the effect of ion concentrations on overall well-being. Negative ion readings by a waterfall average 30,000 per cubic centimetre (perhaps this contributes to the invigorating effects of a shower); in the countryside 1,500 per cubic centimetre; in the average home the level is approximately 100 per cubic centimetre.

Many people with health difficulties such as hay fever, bronchial complaints, asthma and migraines report a marked easing of their condition once the negative ion concentration in their immediate vicinity is raised. Others report the alleviation of problems like fuzzy-headedness, mild headache, catarrh and sinus difficulties when in such an environment.

A range of household ionisers can now be bought which generate negative ions into the home or workplace. Smaller machines are also available for cars and service vehicles. Some work by neutralising any excess of positive ions, as well as generating large numbers of negatively charged ones. These small machines run on mains electricity and can be moved easily from room to room. There are no known side-effects; although a common by-product of ionisers is ozone, the amount they produce is no greater than that found in fresh air. People often let them run through the night in their bedrooms and report improvements in everything from the speed at which they can get off to sleep and the quality of their dreams to a reduction in snoring.

Ionisers are, in a sense, the latest thing, and until some standardisation of reporting is introduced, these claims can not be proved. One thing does seem clear, though; that people with ionisers do report these changes and improvements in their health and feelings of well-being. There is evidence of some of the effects of high levels of negative ions and there is every reason to suppose that redressing any imbalance in local ionisation can have positive health implications.

Substituting natural fibres for synthetics at home and choosing clothing made from cotton, linen, wool, etc., can make a tremendous difference too. Although we cannot all live close to a waterfall or in the middle of a wood, the more we allow nature into our homes and our lives, the better our overall health. (It is also ever-easier to justify a holiday with each new piece of information which proves how greatly the natural world influences our health for the better.)

Finding out more

Friends of the Earth
26-28 Underwood Street
London N1 7JQ
Tel: 071 490 1555

London Ecology Centre
45 Shelton Street
Covent Garden
London WC2H 9HJ
Tel: 071 379 4324

Wholistic Research Company
Bright Haven
Robin's Lane
Lolworth
Cambridge CB3 8HH
Tel: 0954 781074

Further reading

Anna Kruger, *H is for ecoHome*, Gaia Books, 1990.

David Pearson, *The Natural House Book*, Conrad Octopus, 1989.

Jonathon Porritt (ed), *Friends of the Earth Handbook*, Optima, 1987.

IRIDOLOGY

This is a method of diagnosis through careful examination of the condition, colouring and markings of the eyes, sometimes called iris diagnosis.

Iridologists claim to be able to ascertain the health of an individual by the state of their eyes – relating particular divisions of the iris to specific body parts. The iris colour, its shape and markings all point to different aspects of the person's life or parts of the body. An individual's strength of will, structural integrity and the state of their liver can all be seen, using a map which divides the iris into a complex series of circles and divisions.

This method of diagnosis is often used by naturopaths and herbalists, who will take a very close look at the condition of the iris either through shining a light into the eye and using a small magnifying glass or by photographing it. A photograph provides a lasting record and also enables the subject to see the practitioner's findings. Otherwise, they will be noted on a chart of the eye which can then be discussed.

People are often surprised at the amount of detail in their own eyes, and the iridologist will draw attention to the shape of the pupil (it can be flattened in parts by the presence of spinal misalignment), the mixture of colours and the presence of specks or patches of white or other colours.

Nobody really knows how these patterns and colourings are formed, but there seems little doubt that they can be accurate

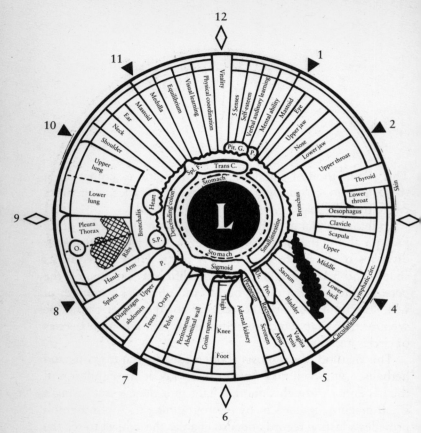

The Iris Map — Left Eye
(mirror image of one's own left eye)

mirrors of health, and this is perhaps best evidenced by noting the changes that can occur in the eye through lifestyle changes and courses of treatment. I first visited an iridologist a day before starting a detoxification programme. When I saw her again, six weeks later, she was able to show me the changes in the clarity of my eyes and the difference in some of the markings. Although many physical changes take some time to

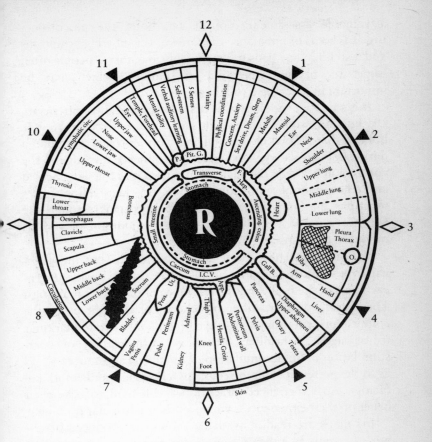

The Iris Map — Right Eye
(mirror image of one's own right eye)

show in the iris, some can be seen within a matter of weeks. Perhaps most useful for preventative care is the fact that general stress and the very early signs of organ distress can be seen, alongside any constitutional or genetic weaknesses or imbalance.

Although this form of diagnosis does not take the place of a case history, it provides a thoroughness and depth that make it a valuable assessment tool. It can point the practitioner towards areas of imbalance that are not yet showing symptoms and also fill in any gaps in the patient's memory – people often forget to mention operations or illnesses which may be important in reaching a full diagnosis.

It is said that iridology was first 'discovered' by a physician, Dr Ignatiev von Peckzely, in the nineteenth century. He noticed that an owl he was nursing with a broken wing had a dark spot in its eye and this led him to investigate the correlation between the changes in this spot as the wing healed and the markings in human eyes. In fact, Hippocrates mentions markings in the eyes, and physicians through the ages have noted being able to see the condition of various organs in this way.

Various maps have been developed, often showing slight variations, but today most people agree on the positioning of each part of the body and the relevance of particular markings. There are, however, different schools of thought as to the colour representations in the eye – some take white markings to be signs of healing, others as an indication of over-stimulation or an accumulation of unnatural substances – and as to the presence of interpretable psychological and emotional factors. An experienced practitioner will tend to base their belief on their experiences, whatever their particular training.

Iris maps are readily available – one is reproduced here – but care must be taken if you decide to take a closer look at your own eyes. They are very light sensitive and can be easily damaged if the light you use is too strong.

Iridology is a diagnostic tool rather than a form of treatment, so how many visits you will need to make to the practitioner and how long a course of treatment takes will vary according to the type of practitioner you choose. As a general rule, once progress is being made with a particular course, an annual check-up and review of overall health is recommended.

Finding out more

British School of Iridology
Dolphin House
6 Gold Street
Saffron Walden
Essex CB10 1EJ

National Council and Register of Iridologists
40 Stockewood Road
Swinton
Bournemouth BH3 7NE
Tel: 0202 529793

Rayid International
408 Dixon Road – SASR
Boulder
Colorado 80302
USA
Tel: (303) 444 4218

Further reading

James and Sheelagh Colton, *Iridology: A Patient's Guide*, Thorsons, 1988.

Dorothy Hall, *Iridology: How the Eyes Reveal your Health and Personality*, Angus and Robertson, 1980.

Adam J. Jackson, *Iridology – A Guide to Iris Analysis and Preventive Health Care*, Optima, 1992.

Bernard Jensen DC ND, *The Science and Practice of Iridology*, BiWorld Publishers, Provo, Utah, 1952.

Henry Lindlahr, *Natural Therapeutics Vol IV Iridiagnosis*, C.W. Daniel, 1975.

JUICING

Fresh fruit and vegetable juices are delicious, quick and easy to prepare, and they are packed full of goodness. Juicing extracts the beneficial minerals, vitamins and essential ingredients from plants and serves them in a tasty, easy and quickly digestible form. Juices have many specific therapeutic uses and can form a valuable addition to an everyday diet.

In some Middle Eastern countries, particularly those where alcohol is forbidden by the religious culture, juicing has been elevated to an art form! There, exotic combinations of fresh mangoes, papaya and kiwi fruit blend together in a delicious alternative to alcohol and carbonated soft drinks (and one that you can reproduce in your own kitchen). In a warmer climate, the need to regulate the body's fluid balance is essential, and fruit and vegetable juices can play an important part in ensuring adequate intake of water. The sense of this lesson can be applied whatever the weather.

A number of good domestic juice extractors are now on the market. Some exciting combinations can be made in a liquidiser, but a proper juicer can soon become an essential and much loved piece of kitchen equipment. Just about anything can be juiced from dandelion leaves (helpful for fluid retention) to the humble but wonderful-tasting carrot (a good source of vitamin A).

The difference between fresh juices and those available commercially is astounding; you can really taste the difference in freshness and flavour and, of course, all the vitamins and minerals are still present in the juice, along with some valuable fibre.

Mixed fruits make a wonderful juice breakfast or a sweet drink at any time of day. Try pineapple and apple as a base and add any other fruit with the exception of bananas. Bananas will not yield juice in most extractors and are best liquidised with a little apple juice or other fruits. During summer the wide range of berries and soft fruits makes for some wonderful combinations, but a simple winter juice of apple, pears and lemon or grapefruit is an all-round winner.

Vegetable juices can be substituted for a meal at any time, and make a tasty and nutritious supplement to any snack. Any variety of raw fresh vegetables can be used, except garlic – the essential oil released is so pungent, its flavour tends to linger in the machine for a long time. Carrot and celery make an excellent base or a refreshing juice on their own. Add lettuce, a little parsley, fennel or whatever else you fancy to make a delicious range of healthy drinks.

Juicing means that the nutrients present in foods can be quickly utilised within the body. They require little energy to process, and enable rapid absorption of the vitamins and minerals they contain. Juices are ideal for providing specific nutrients and allow the digestive system to rest.

An occasional day spent on vegetable juices alone gives the body a rejuvenating fillip – supplying lots of essential nutrients and giving the body a day off from its usual digestive tasks. This frees up all the energy that is normally spent on dealing with the foods we eat, which means it can be used for other valuable jobs in the body.

Juicing also provides an alternative way of obtaining the beneficial properties from plants and herbs.

A handful of young nettles or parsley mixed with other vegetables for juicing can provide the body with much needed iron and both are good skin cleansers. Fifteen drops of juiced mistletoe leaves taken each day is an age-old remedy to increase fertility. (Care must be taken if picking mistletoe leaves because the berries are poisonous.) Adding some fresh red peppers to a juice gives extra vitamin A, and raw beetroot will give the liver a tonic.

Many naturopaths recommend juices for short cleansing diets, or when the body is in need of a rest. They also serve as an excellent introduction to whole foods after any form of fasting. When taking only juices, the stomach has just one kind of food on which to work, and people with health difficulties such as poor absorption can benefit enormously from this form of mono-diet.

A day on freshly juiced apples mixed with live goat's yoghurt is an excellent tonic for many people with digestive difficulties, and a combination of pineapple and apple makes a refreshing cleanser, especially for meat eaters. Mixed cucumber, carrot and lettuce juice can be very helpful for people suffering with mild fluid retention, and the addition of some beetroot, celery or dandelion leaves will help accelerate the process.

Juices are the ideal way to provide nourishment during periods of convalescence and at times when the appetite is low. If used specifically for health purposes, then organically grown produce should really be used. A few years ago I spent just one month on a wholly organic diet and then prepared a juice made from chemically grown fruits. I could taste a number of unpleasant flavours and felt quite sick afterwards. The pesticides and other chemicals present in foods grown this way enter the body much more quickly when taken as part of a juice and those sensitive to such additives should always choose organics.

Finding out more

Incorporated Society of Registered Naturopaths
1 Albemarle Road
The Mount
York YO2 1EN

The Soil Association Ltd
86–88 Colston Street
Bristol
BS1 5BB
Tel: 0272 290661

Further reading

Thorsons, *The Complete Raw Juice Therapy*, 1989.

Bernard Jensen, *Doctor-Patient Handbook*, Bernard Jensen Enterprises, California, 1976.

KINESIOLOGY

Kinesiology, or Applied Kinesiology, was devised by an American chiropractor, Dr George Goodheart, in 1965. It is essentially a system of muscle testing, the results of which can be said to point to any deficiencies in organ function and general health. It was devised as an adjunct to chiropractic work, to correct structural imbalances and as an aid to diagnosis.

The large muscle groups are initially tested for their strength and uniformity of response, and smaller individual muscles may then be tested to pin-point any dysfunction. These are then treated by the use of massage and pressure on specified points which relate to the meridians or energy pathways within the body. Any weaknesses can also point towards nervous impairment resulting from spinal misalignments.

The system is really a synthesis of the best of Eastern tradition (the energy map) and manipulative therapy, with an anatomical base. The muscles which lie on the path that the meridian is said to take through the body are related to the organ which governs that meridian. So, a poor muscle response on the liver meridian as it passes through the shoulder area may point to a lower than normal liver energy, which can be improved through the strengthening of that muscle.

'AK' is nowadays also used for allergy testing on the basis that, if an allergy is present, the body will not be working effectively. This form of testing is used by a number of body-workers and some nutritionists, and a growing number of dentists now use it to assess sensitivity to mercury amalgam fillings.

The classic test is to have the patient stand with one arm extended. The practitioner will pull down on this arm against the patient's resistance and assess its strength. A quantity of a test substance, often chalk or another mineral, will then be held in the patient's other hand while the test is repeated; there should be no change in the response. The substance will then be replaced by a piece of amalgam (or other suspected allergen) while the test is repeated once more. In the case of a sensitivity, the arm will appear much weaker, falling easily under the same pressure which it had just resisted.

These tests can also be used to confirm the benefits of some substances and have been used to demonstrate the positive effects of crystals on the individual's energy. Holding a crystal for a short period of time can be seen to strengthen the test response, without the meridian being worked on at all. This again demonstrates the battery-type effect of quartz and other crystals which can recharge or balance a person.

People are often surprised at the intensity of their response to these seemingly simple techniques, and this is an important factor in confirming their effectiveness. It would be too simple to suggest that the changing response is due totally to psychological factors, or mind over matter, or that changes in effectiveness could occur as the muscle becomes tired. The testing does seem to accurately reflect the body's condition, and most people are convinced of that after just one try.

AK muscle testing can also be used to check for vitamin and mineral deficiencies. The patient touches a body part relating to the nutrient with one hand, while the other arm is tested. The need for B vitamins, for example, can be measured with the patient touching the tip of their tongue.

Since its inception, AK has branched further into behavioural kinesiology (created by John Diamond to concentrate on environmental and lifestyle factors) and **Touch for Health**.

Cross Crawling is a wonderfully invigorating kinesiology exercise. It has been seen to improve co-ordination between the right and left hemispheres of the brain and as such has proved important in the treatment of children with impaired development. Its application for adults is as a refreshing, enlivening exercise, and one that can improve concentration and relieve weariness.

Stand upright with feet shoulder width apart and begin to 'march' on the spot. Lift the knees quite high and bring them slightly in towards the midline with each lift, extending them back to their original place as you put your feet down.

Swing your left arm across your body as your right knee comes up and back as your right foot is replaced. Swing your right arm across your body as your left knee comes up and back as your left foot is replaced. This is a complicated thing to describe in words, but is very simple to do. Imagine yourself wanting to cross a midline point in your body with both your upper and lower limbs. To keep a nice rhythm, you use your right arm with your left leg.

This arm swings across the body

This leg swings across the body

Behavioural kinesiology has added an emotional aspect to the treatment and has proved a valuable form of testing for environmental allergies.

Touch for health was devised by John F. Thie for use by the lay person. He intended its use to provide the opportunity for families to share a new kind of touching – one that is healing rather than invasive or sexual.

Touch for health is a simplified form of AK and one that can easily be used by individuals in their own homes. It forms the basis for the muscle testing described above, and includes straightforward forms of treatment and assessment. Touch for Health also includes a more energetic focus and contains many techniques to address specific energy imbalances.

Finding out more

Association for of Systematic Kinesiology
39 Browns Road
Surbiton
Surrey KT5 8ST
Tel: 081 399 3215

Touch for Health Foundation
1174 North Lake Avenue
Pasedena
California 91104-3797
USA
Tel: (818) 794 1181

Further reading

John F. Thie, *Touch for Health: A new approach to restoring our natural energies*, D.C. DeVorss and Company, Marina del Rey, California, 1973.

LEADING EDGE THERAPIES

Therapeutic Touch · Exercise trends · Neuro-Linguistic Programming · Psycho-Neuroimmunology

There are many therapies at the leading edge of natural healthcare. Pushing back perceived boundaries, the themes of personal development and individual growth lend themselves to new interpretation. The concept of self-responsibility in health is not new, yet the degree to which we are able to embrace it changes with each new decade and, on an individual level, with each successive personal revelation.

Many established therapies give rise to new approaches, as practitioners include their personal attributes and develop their own synthesis of techniques. In this respect, every responsible natural healthcare practitioner is at the leading edge of their profession.

Blends of different skills and philosophies give rise to new schools of thought, too, as in the development of **Therapeutic Touch,** which was designed in 1975 for non-psychics who had the desire to heal. This was developed by Dolores Krieger, an American nurse, and she has now trained many others in this work which is rapidly gaining in popularity both in the United States and across the world.

Exercise, another important facet of a healthy lifestyle, has seen many changes over the years. From the early popularity of calasthenic-based trainings, the 'burn', aerobics, and yoga as exercise have today been surpassed by cardiac funk (a low-impact, full-body aerobic workout, that is now gaining converts from the general public and health experts alike), and aquaerobics. The concept of exercise in water is not new, but the recognition of the benefits of working against natural resistance is here combined with current knowledge of the body's need for sustained aerobic work.

At the forefront of psychotherapeutics, **Neuro-linguistic Programming** is gaining wide acclaim, offering a radically new way of interpreting our motivations and drives. NLP was born out of observations of the success of three therapists – Virginia Satir, Milton Erickson and Fritz Perls. They each used different styles of therapy and were all extremely successful. The factors that were common to each of their practices were isolated and developed to form the basis for NLP.

Providing individuals and therapists with new insights into the differing frames of reference that we all use, NLP sessions extend the educative aspect of the work to the client. Used mainly as a tool for potentially dynamic personal change, these techniques start by defining the mode of recall with which the individual feels most comfortable: some of us rely on visual memory, others rely on auditory memory, etc. Assessments of eye movements, pupil size and direction of gaze also provide clues as to the importance of specific memories, and where we store them – for instance as a personal reflection, something learned or an inspired thought.

Ancient philosophy suggests that much dispute is born of miscommunication. NLP provides many ways in which the miscommunication between individuals, partners and groups may be identified, and offers techniques for reducing this common occurrence. The techniques are easy to learn and put into practice, and most practitioners will include in their sessions instruction on those skills which are likely to be most useful. NLP provides a quick and useful way of managing change and, as well as its long-term usefulness, can work very effectively with immediate issues.

An area of research that is currently exciting many allopathic practitioners is **Psycho-Neuroimmunology.** In the USA the connections between how we feel emotionally and how our bodies work are being investigated, and proven! Researchers have been able to measure in a scientific way the changes that occur in the immune systems of individuals who have been exposed to emotional trauma or who are grieving. It has been found that the reproduction of some specific cells which help rid the body of invaders, and also those which are involved in repressing tumour activity, is slowed down. Groups of individuals whose stress levels are high – those facing the pressures of work deadlines, final exams, caring for sick or elderly relatives, for example – have more sluggish immune systems which do not rise to the challenge of disease control as quickly or ably as those experiencing lower levels of stress. It seems that when people feel emotionally depressed or are experiencing negative physical *or* emotional states, the way their bodies work is also depressed. It is being proposed that psychological factors are more influential in morbidity than smoking, obesity, blood pressure or exercise.

The concept, for instance, that psychological stress may be as important a contributor to a smoker's health as physiological stress is a radical one. I wonder if health warnings on cigarette packs might one day read: 'Warning – Stop and think *why* you are reaching for that cigarette.'

At least this is encouraging more people to recognise the integrity of the human individual – an entity comprising feelings and emotions that are intrinsic to a physical manifestation. Once again, though, we see this branch of science taking the wisdom from natural healthcare but denying the therapy. Once this connection is satisfactorily verified, perhaps allopathic medicine will do more to embrace a view of the human organism that is more than just a sum of disassociated parts.

As this book is being written, a Bill is being prepared for the British Parliament that could take osteopathy into the National Health Service. This would place osteopaths in the same professional ranks as doctors and dentists – a first for alternative medicine. Nobody can say at this stage what may come of this, but there seem to be two main possibilities: osteopathy could be slotted in to the hospital services as part of the physiotherapy department; or, bearing in mind the enormous practical and philosophical difficulties of such an idea, this could herald the beginning of alternative therapies being recognised in their own right as areas of speciality.

This opens up an entirely new vision of the future; one in which individuals' responsibility for their own healthcare could be legitimately recognised, and they could make informed choices independent of cultural mores or personal finances.

Finding out more

British Touch for Health Association
8 Railey Mews
London NW5 2PA
Tel: 071 482 0698

UK Training Centre for NLP
11 Buckland Crescent
Hampstead
London NW3
Tel: 071 483 2384

Further reading

R.Bandler and J. Frinder, *Frogs into Princes*, Real People Press, 1978.

James P. Carse, *Finite and Infinite Games*, Penguin, 1986.

Dolores Krieger PhD RN, *Therapeutic Touch: How to Use Your Hands to Help and Heal*, Prentice Hall, 1979.

Janet Macrae, *Therapeutic Touch: A Practical Guide*, Penguin, 1990.

Eric Robbie, *What is NLP?*, self-published, 1989. Available in specialist bookshops.

Robert Anton Wilson, *Prometheus Rising*, Falcon Press, 1983.

MANIPULATIVE THERAPIES

Osteopathy · Chiropractic · McTimoney

Osteopathy is an important aspect of naturopathy, adding an important, physically changing therapy to the simple philosophies of nature cure. Devised by an American, Andrew Taylor Still in 1874, it is a method of directly addressing structural difficulties and influencing the rest of the body. Some form of physical manipulation has been used for centuries, seen in ancient American Indian hieroglyphs, forming part of Hippocrates' teachings and even impressing Captain Cook in the eighteenth century during his travels to Tahiti.

The spine is comprised of a number of separate bones linked together to provide a solid protection for the spinal cord. There are seven bones or vertebrae in the neck, or cervical region, twelve in the upper and mid-back (thoracic area), and five in the low back (lumbar spine) before reaching the sacrum and coccyx or tail bone. The size and shape of the bones varies from one region to another and the joints between all these different-shaped bones are designed to enable full movement in a range of different directions (the direction of movement changing from one area to another).

Obviously, problems can occur if there is bad posture or incorrect use, when the muscles can place stresses on these joints, or if there is any sudden exertion or accident. Any of these things can cause back pain, but perhaps more important is their effect on other areas of the body.

In the vicinity of the joint is a space for nerves to leave the protection of the spinal cord and travel to the organs and areas of the body that they supply. These nerves carry the stimuli which enable the body to work and also relay messages back to the brain. If there is irritation or dysfunction in this key area around the vertebral joint, then the messages relayed by the nerves may become impaired.

Osteopaths are trained to assess the structural integrity of the spine and the other joints of the body. They do this through observing movement restrictions and areas of immobility and through palpation or touch.

After your history has been given, and the details of any specific complaint you may have, the practitioner will ask you to undress as far as your underwear to allow a proper look at your back. If the problem is in another body part, the osteopath will check your spine anyway. Some practitioners will provide gowns, like those you will find at a hospital, which can be opened down the back.

First of all you will be asked to carry out a range of active movements, which the practitioner will observe – like walking up and down, bending, and turning your head. You will then be taken through a range of passive movements (these require no muscular effort, rather the practitioner will move your body for you).

A number of neurological tests and an assessment of muscle condition will follow and the practitioner will then investigate the degree of movement between each separate vertebra. This is done by placing a light hand pressure on each vertebra in turn whilst moving or mobilising those on either side of it.

All of this takes place with the patient either seated or lying down and should cause no pain, although some slight discomfort may be felt if the osteopath finds an area with a problem or lesion. At this stage a diagnosis can be made, and the treatment may stop while the osteopath informs the patient of their findings and explains what is to happen next.

If the practitioner has found an area of misplacement (a lesion or sometimes called subluxation) they are likely to manipulate it back into position. To do this, the body is placed in a position enabling it to be used as a long lever, with the area of lesion at the fulcrum. This may entail twisting the body or putting it into strange positions to set up the manipulation, which is carried out speedily and, usually, painlessly. Sometimes the manipulation will involve a thrust directly onto the lesioned vertebrae, without moving the body as a whole. When this takes place a clunk or click sound may be heard, usually accompanied by instant feelings of relief. When the vertebrae in the neck are manipulated this clunking sound appears to be much louder, but it is not at all dangerous.

The osteopath may make a number of manipulations in different areas of the body during a treatment, and may also demonstrate specific exercises to maintain mobility throughout the area. These should be repeated, as prescribed, and will be followed up in subsequent sessions. The first appointment will usually last for an hour, if the practitioner is also a naturopath, or thirty to forty-five minutes if not. Subsequent visits vary from twenty minutes to an hour.

Obviously, there are some people who should not be manipulated in such a way, and some health concerns that preclude this form of treatment − post-menopausal women who are at risk of osteoporosis (a thinning of the bone mass); those with a history of tuberculosis; and anyone in acute pain are a few examples. An osteopath will determine what form of treatment is advisable when they take the case history.

Another form of manipulative therapy is **Chiropractic**. This is the main choice in the USA, and is becoming more popular throughout Europe. Chiropractors work in a very similar way to osteopaths with a few important distinctions. They rely almost exclusively on X-rays for diagnosis, whereas osteopaths tend to use them as a back-up measure to confirm any findings. These can be taken quickly because many chiropractors have X-ray equipment at their practice. The benefits of this thorough approach need to be balanced against the exposure to radiation.

Because chiropractors spend much less time actually examining the patient, some appointments can be completed in ten minutes. The other main difference is in the style of manipulation. Chiropractors tend to prefer more direct thrusts, while osteopaths prefer 'long-lever' techniques. There is much debate as to which is easier for the patient, but an important point is that neither is likely to cause any degree of pain or tissue damage. Direct thrusts involve placing pressure on the vertebrae, and using a quick, specific push to reposition it. Long-lever techniques involve positioning the body so that the vertebra is encouraged to right itself, and will require minimal force from the practitioner to complete the repositioning.

The technique of applied kinesiology was originated by an American chiropractor, Dr George Goodheart, in 1965. This now forms a part of many chiropractic treatments, although there also exist a number of practitioners working solely with this therapy (see Applied Kinesiology page 134).

Another branch of chiropractic called **McTimoney** technique has recently evolved. I understand this concentrates on a more widespread approach to manipulation, incorporating some of the best chiropractic techniques with osteopathic concepts to develop a useful form of bodywork which is gentle on the body.

Osteopaths can now be found at a few hospitals, where their treatments are available on the National Health Service. These are pilot schemes and as yet the government has no plans to extend their availability. Both osteopaths and chiropractors work at natural health clinics and in private practice, and some also advertise in the Yellow Pages. There are fewer McTimoney practitioners because the therapy is still relatively new, but they clearly differentiate themselves as McTimoney chiropractors and so are relatively easy to find.

Manipulative therapists may suggest specific exercises to mobilise parts of the spine or to strengthen certain muscle groups that are important for the maintenance of good posture.

This is a particularly good exercise for strengthening and stretching the back and neck and also gives the lymphatic system a boost.

Sit upright on a chair with both feet flat on the floor. Slowly begin to lower your chin down on to your chest and raise your arms to interlock your fingers just behind the crown of your head. Gently lower your hands on to your head and let their weight bring your head down lower. Slowly relax the arms and your elbows will move down and towards each other in front of you; the weight of your arms drawing your head down still further. You should be able to feel the stretch in your neck and upper back; if you are not generally active, or if there are any areas of immobility in your spine, you may feel the stretch right down to your tail bone or sacrum.

Hold this position for ten to twenty breaths and then very slowly reverse the process: slowly lifting your elbows and raising your hands and then last of all your head.

Next let your head move slowly backwards, making sure that your back is still straight. Do not stretch your head back, just let it reach the point where you begin to feel the muscles at the front of your neck start to tighten. Jut your chin up and out past your upper teeth and feel the stretch down into your sternum or chest bone.

Hold this position for ten to twenty breaths and then slowly lift your head back up to an upright position.

Finding out more

British Naturopathic and Osteopathic Association
6 Netherhall Gardens
London NW3 5RR
Tel: 071 435 8728

British Osteopathic Association
8-19 Boston Place
London NW1 6QH
Tel: 071 262 5250

Natural Therapeutic and Osteopathic Society
14 Marford Road
Wheathampstead
Herts AL4 8AS
Tel: 058283 3950

British Chiropractic Association
Premier House
Greycoat Place
London SW1P 1SB
Tel: 071 222 8866

Chiropractic Advancement Association
56 Barnes Crescent
Wimborne
Dorset BH21 2AZ

Institute of Pure Chiropractic (this is McTimoney!)
14 Park End Street
Oxford OH1 1HH

Scottish Chiropractic Association
30 Roseburn Place
Edinburgh
EH12 5NX
Tel: 031 346 7500

Further reading

Susan Moore, *Chiropractic*, Optima, 1988.

Stephen Sandler, *Osteopathy*, Optima, 1987.

MASSAGE THERAPY

Massage has been defined as 'treatment of the muscles using rubbing or kneading'. Anyone who has received a good massage can tell of the many different levels on which they felt cared for and treated. This hands-on method of working on the whole body can be used to treat muscle soreness and stiffness, but it can also do a lot more than that.

Massage techniques can be used to help individuals with specific complaints ranging from asthma and bronchitis to menstrual pain. They can be incorporated into any stress management plan for the total relaxation they help to engender, and can also be used to address a number of joint problems. They can aid suppleness in the body by breaking down fluid retention, fatty deposits and releasing areas of immobility. Massage can also be used to access and aid in the resolution of emotional issues. Most often, though, it is seen as a treat.

On a physical level, a general massage will improve lymphatic drainage, increase overall circulation, stimulate the nervous system and soothe the skin. It can provide an enormous energy boost, whilst containing that in an easy, relaxed way. Massage can also improve communication between mind and body, and can be a tremendous aid to anybody seeking an increased physical awareness.

Most massage therapists work at health clinics and sports facilities, although some will also visit your home. The initial session will begin with the taking of a short health history. The therapist will also want to know about any specific aches and pains and whether there are any 'trouble-spots'. We all tend to hold tensions somewhere in the body, the commonest sites are the shoulders, low back and stomach – these are the places that ache or get uncomfortably tight when we are stressed. If you are not aware of any particular tensions, the therapist will soon find what areas need to be worked on once the massage begins.

The therapy room might feel unusually warm to begin with, but this is important to ensure full relaxation when you are being massaged. Lying still (with the presence of oil or cream on your skin) can make you feel slightly colder than normal, and if the room is not to be warmer than usual, your muscles are likely to tense – this would undo many of the beneficial effects of the treatment.

Some people undress completely to receive a massage, others leave on their underwear. The therapist will be quite used to working with all sorts of bodies, so modesty need not be an issue – it is important to do whatever will feel most comfortable for you. Any body parts not being worked on will be covered with a towel or blanket, and this helps with the question of modesty as well as providing additional warmth.

You can elect to have just a back or a neck and shoulder massage if this is what you would prefer, although a full treatment is most beneficial. A full body massage usually begins with a person lying on their tummy on the treatment couch, while the therapist begins work on their back. Some form of cream is most often used, although some therapists prefer to use oils. (See Aromatherapy for the use of essential oils.) One of the most wonderful aspects of this type of work is that, however bright or quick-thinking you may be, it is impossible to keep track of the different techniques and pressure strokes that the therapist will use. There really is no option, then, but just to concentrate on relaxing and enjoying the pleasurable feelings. Being able to receive that amount of

care in such a relaxed and secure environment is a tremendously enriching experience.

Touch has to be one of our most underused senses – usually
this degree of tactile nourishment only takes place between
mother and baby or between lovers. Perhaps this is one of the
reasons why the word is used as a misnomer by escort agencies
and the like. Nothing could be further from the truth for
massage therapy, however, and this is why many female
therapists will only work on other women. Although massage
therapy has nothing to do with sex or sexual massage, many
women find it easier to relax in this way with another woman.

During a treatment, the legs and neck will also be worked
on before turning the client or patient over and covering the
front of the legs, the arms and hands, neck, shoulders and face.
Your abdomen and chest seem to be an optional extra – most
therapists will ask you if you want these areas to be treated.

Although using a similar range of techniques – stroking,
percussion, kneading, pummelling, etc. – each massage therapist will develop their own style, so the feelings and the
treatment will vary from one practitioner to another. There are
also areas of specialty – some therapists concentrate on sports
or remedial massage, others on relaxation or on the beauti-
fying aspects of improving skin tone and texture (partly from
all that lovely cream or oil). Massage can also assist weight
reduction by stimulating the lymphatic system and helping to
break down fatty tissue. It is important to establish what type
of massage you want – relaxation, for example, or to help with
a training injury.

Many healers also use massage, and concentrate on the
more energetic aspects of the treatment. Intuitive massage
therapists allow themselves to be guided to areas of tension by
the way the client's body feels, rather than by following any
strict anatomical pattern.

After a treatment, there is usually time to just lie still and
appreciate the wonderful, warm feelings of deep physical

relaxation. The therapist will be busy washing their hands and writing up your notes and may even leave you alone for a while to gather your thoughts before you need to dress again. Many clinics and health centres have shower facilities which you can use after a treatment, but it is also nice not to have to do anything other than hold onto those positive feelings. Those lucky enough to find a therapist who will visit at home can, of course, remain totally relaxed for as long as they wish.

Some massage oils can stain certain fabrics (particularly poly-cottons) so you may want to have a change of clothing with you, but your skin will have absorbed most of the cream or oil that was used.

Massage therapy courses are available at many adult education centres and at health clinics. It is very easy, though, to begin massaging yourself and friends or family without any formal training. A good shoulder rub can be wonderful at the end of a busy day, and it is easy to feel any tight spots even through layers of clothing. Children love being massaged and baby massage is a wonderfully soothing experience for both baby and adult.

You can massage yourself easily anywhere except on the back. This is a lovely way to end the day, or as an after-bath treat. Simply use some cream body lotion or oil and begin by gently stroking whichever body part you are working on. Follow the contours of your skin closely with your hands, and vary the pressure and the length of each stroke. Simple kneading movements can be made by pressing down with your hands, and knuckles can be used on fleshy areas and on the soles of the feet. If you have a professional massage you may well pick up some tips for other techniques, but simply covering yourself with your own loving, caring touch can be remarkably therapeutic.

Finding out more

The Churchill Centre
22 Montagu Street
London W1H 1TB
Tel: 071 402 9475

Clare Maxwell-Hudson School of Massage
87 Dartmouth Road
London NW2 4ER
Tel: 081 450 6494

The Northern Institute of Massage
100 Waterloo Road
Blackpool
Lancashire FY4 1AW
Tel: 0253 403548

Further reading

George Downing, *The Massage Book*, Arkana, 1972.

Roberta deLong Miller, *Psychic Massage*, Harper & Row.

MEDITATION

Meditation is the practice of stilling the conscious mind and allowing a 'free space'; a time of renewal and rejuvenation for the body and mind.

Meditation takes many forms, and the different schools and philosophies advocate a variety of techniques for attaining this state. It is one of the best natural therapies. Through meditation we can approach and embrace higher levels of awareness. The conscious mind may then interpret the new experience and the whole person benefits.

Some people use meditation as a form of relaxation; others to achieve 'time off' from physical and mental concerns. It can also be a powerful aid to personal growth and a deeply spiritual experience.

One technique is to train the mind systematically to be aware of different areas of the body and to recognise any local stresses. These can be consciously relaxed and the mind is then free to float, allowing the body to recharge itself. This takes conventional relaxation skills one step further in that the time spent once physical relaxation is achieved is perhaps the most valuable of all.

Active meditation is a unique method of problem solving. The problem or question to be asked is repeated over and over again either silently or out loud, and this serves to focus the individual's resources almost entirely. The repeating can be continued for a day or longer – it is important that there should be no other claims on the person's attention, so time is often a limiting factor. Suddenly, there seems to come a point when, almost like the waters of a river breaking through a surface covering of ice, the tension of holding the thought becomes almost unbearable and an answer bubbles up from somewhere deep inside. Such moments of personal revelation can be deeply inspiring, renewing our confidence in our own inner source of wisdom.

Those following a guru or the teachings of a spiritual leader will often meditate with the guru's photograph, or whilst listening to the sound of their voice. This facilitates a sense of connection with their teacher and serves as a reminder of their presence or vibrations. Many gurus, in keeping with their Indian and Eastern traditions, advocate a regular practice of meditation as part of any spiritual journey or preparation for enlightenment.

The reasoning behind this is based on the assumption that we all have our own unique path to follow – our own star. Only by reinforcing the connection with our own inner motivations and wisdom can we be true to ourselves and fulfil our own promise or destiny. More immediately, this awareness of our inner selves helps us to act in ways that are right or appropriate for us. In a busy world of conflicting demands and influences, meditation can support individual integrity and clarify choices.

It is from a feeling of knowledge of and security within ourselves that we may reach out and embrace other experiences. Meditation can therefore be centred around uniting us with universal principles such as love or peace. Within the framework of a teaching or religion, the Buddha-energy or Christ-energy may be held as a model for that experience. An important point is that the focus here is on the awareness of a quality or archetype that may be touched to expand our consciousness.

Meditation is not a way of escaping from reality, although it is a remarkable way of transcending our everyday experiences and reconnecting with our higher selves. The feeling can be described as truly 'out of this world', although some people feel that they reach to a place deep within themselves, whereas others sense a place beyond their usual frames of reference.

Chants and mantras are often used to aid meditation; either as something to occupy the mind and, through repetition, to seduce it into stillness; or for the harmonic or vibration of the sound itself. Perhaps the most well known of these is 'OHM'. This is repeated slowly, starting with a full breath, and feeling the belly of the 'O' coming from a place below the diaphragm. The sound then rises, along with the chanter's energy, through the body and into the upper part of the head by the time the 'M' is reached.

Other techniques include fixing the attention on a visual image such as a simple shape in a primary colour, a red circle for example. This is stared at for some time until the image is retained in the mind when the eyes are closed. This, too, serves as something on which to concentrate the mind until a deeper relaxation is achieved. A similar image is that of an imaginary line – just a straight line, that extends out in front of you. With closed eyes, this line can be followed, leading you out of your current consciousness or state of awareness.

A number of psychics use a candle flame for another form of meditation which actually develops their seeing sense or visual perception skills. Focusing on the flame, they work to alter its colour – changing it through the colours of the rainbow before reverting to seeing it as it is. The symbol of a flower bud can be used in a similar way – seeing it unfold, close, change colours, etc. Many psychics find themselves free to experience a meditative state whilst focusing their psychic energies in this way.

Some people seem to be able to achieve meditation very easily, or whenever they want to. For others, a regular practice is an important part of the learning process. All the techniques are really just means to an end, so one or more can be used, or they can all be experimented with before finding a way that works best.

It is usually best to begin in a comfortable sitting position, making sure that you are warm enough, and that there are not likely to be any interruptions. The burning of incense can encourage feelings of restfulness and is also said to remind us of spirit energy in the transformation from the matter of the cone, granules or sticks, through flame, to something that affects us (the smell) but that we can neither see nor touch.

Initially, when sitting silently, the mind has a tendency to review all sorts of things. Memories and ideas seem to flood the thoughts and it is easy to follow any one of them. The aim of meditation is not to pay these mental workings any notice, rather to centre the attention in another place – one that will not be influenced by the passing thoughts, but is able just to let them come and go. The position of onlooker is cultivated, one that is non-judgemental, yet strong enough not to be seduced from its purpose.

Half-an-hour or twenty minutes is a good time to set aside for this practice. An alarm clock can be used to mark the end of the meditation, but a gentler, less jarring method would be better; ideally, just trusting to an inner clock that will allow you to remain in meditation for just as long as you need.

Many Buddhist centres teach classes in meditation, and they can also be found at a number of adult education centres. This simple practice is a powerful way of uniting body and mind and encouraging awareness of our subtle or energetic nature. It can also be a reminder of a time when we were not separate from the world; a reuniting with the world of spirit or the source.

Finding out more

London Soto Zen Group
c/o Duncan Sellers
23 Westbere Road
London NW2
Tel: 071 794 3109

London Zen Society
10 Belmont Street
London NW1
Tel: 071 485 9576

RIGPA Fellowship
44 St Paul's Crescent
Camden Town
London NW1 9TN
Tel: 071 485 4342

School of Meditation
158 Holland Park Avenue
London W11 4UH
Tel: 071 603 6116

NATUROPATHY OR NATURAL THERAPEUTICS

Nature cure, naturopathy and natural therapeutics are all terms adopted to designate a system of natural healing; natural in the sense that it must be in accordance with natural law. In natural law, we look at natural or normal basic behavioural patterns, e.g. nutrition; reproduction; outdoor habit (contact with fresh air, sun, etc.); contact with water, soil and other organisms; exercise, play and sleeping patterns.

There is a large range of therapies considered 'natural', including dietary therapy, massage, neuromuscular technique, osteopathy and other bodywork, hydrotherapy, clay therapy, the use of herbs, exercise and counselling – all the therapies covered in this book, in fact. Most naturopathic trainings cover all of these topics, although the emphasis changes according to different schools of thought – some concentrating on a wide knowledge of the many available treatment forms, others concentrating on one or two modalities and an understanding of the others.

One turn-of-the-century catechism of nature cure defined it as 'A system of the person building in harmony with the constructive principle in nature, on the physical, mental and moral planes of being.' Heavy with the language of that time, this definition does at least give an example of the comprehensive scope of natural therapy.

By the 1960s a British naturopathic association had developed the following outline: 'Nature cure is a philosophic concept on which naturopathy is founded. This concept embraces a belief in and a full appreciation of the self-regulating, self-adjusting and self-healing ability of the human organism, scientifically termed homoeostasis.

'Naturopathy is the professional practice of those therapies based upon the nature cure concept which are directed towards the releasing of the inherent healing force, therefore aiding in the restoration of the homoeostatic equilibrium and in the reversal of the disease process.'

So, the naturopath's motto is 'only nature heals', and the work is in finding ways to facilitate that healing in appropriate and non-interventionist ways; in finding ways to support the body's own healing process, the primary objective of naturopathy is not just to cure, but to educate the patient to live in harmony with their body's unique recipe.

All practising naturopaths will develop their own synthesis of techniques for working with the body's own vitality, although they will all cover three basic areas – body systems, structure and a counselling aspect. One of the most common medley of therapies is naturopathic dietary therapy and lifestyle advice, osteopathy or massage, and some form of counselling.

There are, of course, purists in the naturopathic world, as there are in any other aspect of life. Some would consider the use of vitamin supplements and herbs as unnatural, and at the other end of the spectrum there are those who include interventionist forms of treatment such as acupuncture as part of their treatment plans.

A visit to a naturopath begins with the taking of a comprehensive case history. The practitioner will want to know about your current lifestyle, relationships and feelings as well as your health history. The illnesses and feelings you had as a child, and some details of your parents' health will add important building blocks to the overall picture of your own vitality and constitution – the ways your body copes with disease and how quickly you recover. Any operations, surgical removals (tonsils, appendix, etc.), immunisations, allergies and broken bones will also help the diagnosis.

Pharmaceuticals often block the body's own ability to cope, so particular attention will be paid to any medicines you are currently taking or courses of drugs taken in the past. (Close to 98 per cent of all prescription drugs have negative side effects, 50 per cent of prescriptions are solely to suppress symptoms, and a recent study showed 48% of antibiotic courses prescribed in the last year in the UK (1991) to have been both unnecessary *and* ineffective!)

Many naturopaths will ask you to keep a diet diary for a few days prior to your first visit, to get an idea of your eating habits and help with assessing your nutritional status. (See Diet Therapy). The consultation may also include some form of structural assessment, usually from an osteopathic viewpoint. This is particularly relevant in the presence of back pain, general aches and pains or problems in a particular area of the body. Routine tests like blood pressure and pulse rate may also be carried out.

Even if you visit a naturopath with a specific health complaint, a full investigation will be made of your overall health because naturopaths maintain that illnesses do not occur in isolation; the whole person is involved. There is no point in treating a symptom without finding and treating the underlying cause. This may mean that the treatment for a stomach ulcer would involve making dietary changes, taking herbs or supplements, learning some form of relaxation technique and perhaps doing some counselling – depending on what caused the ulcer to occur in the first place. In this respect, naturopaths work as primary care providers, fulfilling the role of a natural GP. They can help with acute situations such as flu and infections as well as more long-term conditions like arthritis and recurring complaints.

Naturopathy takes a distinct view of disease – placing importance on the individual's resistance and ability to overcome health difficulties, rather than on the nature of an infecting organism. Symptoms are often seen as the body's attempt to increase elimination and overcome the disease itself, or as signs pointing to the area of the real problem. A cold might well be a good sign of increased resilience on the part of the mucous membraines – particularly if it occurs after giving up smoking, for instance, when the body will need to expel a number of toxins that have accumulated in the lungs and bronchi. A skin complaint may point to a sluggish bowel condition; when the bowel is not functioning well, stresses are placed on the body's other eliminative routes and organs – the kidneys, lungs, liver and skin. Skill is needed to determine whether the symptoms are a positive sign to be encouraged – a healing crisis – as distinct from a situation in need of support – a disease crisis.

After a full diagnosis has been made, the naturopath will draw on a wide variety of treatments to provide the best possible care in resolving the symptoms and improving the constitution. This usually entails some work on the part of the patient, who will need to be actively involved in their own healthcare. In aiming to give individuals the responsibility for their own health, the practitioner's role is most often as advisor – suggesting diets, providing herbs, initiating new lines of thought or exercise plans. Even the more physically based aspects of a treatment, e.g. an osteopathic adjustment, may require a commitment from the patient in terms of learning how to lift correctly or maintaining an easy posture if the problem is not to recur.

Once a course of treatment is underway, the naturopath may refer you to other therapists – for some massage for example – and continue as a co-ordinator or central focus for your ongoing health.

Most naturopaths will develop their own areas of specialisation, so this is worth asking about at the initial consultation. Some may concentrate on the links between mind and body, for instance, focusing on an integrated view and being able to offer psychological counselling as a mainstay of the treatment. Others may rely more on constitutional change, using herbs, diet and hydrotherapy to restore and maintain health.

Treatments usually last an hour, although the initial consultation may last longer. Courses of treatment vary in length although most naturopaths will continue to fulfil a 'GP-type' function, treating ongoing and changing health considerations as they occur.

Finding out more

British Naturopathic Association
6 Netherhall Gardens
London NW3 5RR
Tel: 071 435 6464

Incorporated Society of British Naturopaths
Kingston
The Coach House
293 Gilmerton Road
Edinburgh EH16 5UQ
Tel: 031 664 3435

Incorporated Society of Registered Naturopaths
1 Albermarle Road
The Mount
York
YO2 1EN

Further reading

Judy Jacka, *A-Z of Natural Therapies*, Lothian Press, Australia, 1988.

Bernard Jensen, *Nature Has A Remedy*, Bernard Jensen Enterprises, California, 1982.

Henry Lindlahr, *Natural Therapeutics*, C.W. Daniel, 1975.

Michael Murray and Joseph Pizzorno, *Encyclopaedia of Natural Medicine*, Optima, 1989.

Ross Trattler ND DO, *Better Health through Natural Healing*, Thorsons, 1987.

OUTDOOR CONTACT

As we become more insulated against the elements in our sturdy homes and hectic lifestyles, it becomes ever easier to lose contact with nature. This even though the natural world still governs our lives through the seasons, the daily cycle of light and dark and the growth of all living things.

Our bodies and emotions are still tuned to a natural clock; influenced by the seasons and in need of contact with the elements. After a day spent indoors, we'll often use the need for fresh air as an excuse to go for a short walk, or to stand in the garden for a while. Yet opening a window would provide the fresh air. What we really feel we need, and often do not know how to express because it is such an instinctive drive, is contact with 'the great outdoors' – to move freely and see nature, perhaps walk on some soil, feel the wind move us, or the sun's touch, or to gaze at the stars. We become unhealthy in body and spirit if deprived of such contact for long.

Many a gardener can tell of the magic of working with soil and of feeling close to other growing things. There is an amazing sensation to be had walking barefoot on clean grass – one can really feel in touch with the planet with which we live. I once read that if topsoil were the equivalent of our protective layer of skin, then grass would be the hair of the giant organism, Earth. This image has stayed with me and, although very romantic, it is an amazing thought to be caressing the

Earth's tresses every time we reach down and touch a patch of grass.

When sunlight touches the skin we can produce vitamin D – essential for health. When we are in natural surroundings, particularly in the presence of moving water, we are bathed in life-enhancing negative ions. Feeling the whisper of a gentle breeze touch our skin, millions of nerve endings are gently stimulated. It is hard to resist the native American teachings that we are all part of the Great Spirit – ourselves and all living things, and Grandmother Earth and Grandfather Sky.

The quality of the air we breathe is so important. We need fresh, clean air for our lungs, so that oxygen can be carried by the blood to every area of the body. Every cell has its own cycle of renewal – it breaks down and is then rebuilt according to its innate sense of timing. Oxygen is an important building block in this process, and the construction of healthy, non-malignant cells relies on oxygen, amongst other things, being available in the right amount. When the air we breathe is polluted, instead of large amounts of oxygen, we provide our bodies with lead, carbon monoxide and a whole host of other noxious and dangerous substances.

As our lungs become polluted, they are less able to achieve the important gaseous exchange which is necessary to prevent a build-up of carbon oxide in the system. The lungs play a vital role as one of the body's main routes of elimination, and any under-functioning here places increased pressure on the rest of the body.

In cities throughout the world, incidences of breathing difficulties and lung disorders increase in line with elevated air pollution levels. Asthma and a wide cross section of allergic reactions and minor immune system dysfunctions occur with increasing regularity as the quality of the air deteriorates.

Trees are the answer – increasing the oxygen content of air faster and more efficiently than anything else. Sadly, as we destroy the rainforests and other woodland areas across the world, we point towards our own destruction. On a more local level, tree-lined avenues, parks and woodlands are really the only places to take exercise or walks.

The ability to breathe fresh, clean air is a basic human need. When we exercise, one of the purposes is to increase the amount of oxygen we take in. It isn't necessary to take large gulps of fresh air – just breathing normally should supply all the oxygen you need, and the simplest of activities will speed up your intake. Walking is one of the best all-round exercises you can do; it is a gentle work out for the whole body, exercising most muscles and improving abdominal tone. Walking gradually increases your oxygen needs and your lungs' ability, thereby improving general fitness. Increasing oxygen requirement whilst walking along busy roads, or in other heavily polluted areas simply increases the rate of poisoning you will experience.

A regular intake of fresh air is a necessary part of all-round good health, and it is vital that this air is clean and good. Many of us live in towns and cities, or close to the motorways which criss-cross much of the countryside, or to industrial centres. All these situations create a special need for fresh air and it is well worth searching out areas that will provide this.

Because this issue is vital, many people, once they have started to enjoy the pleasures of more outdoor contact, feel that they have a responsibility to campaign in some way for anti-pollution legislation, local clean-air campaigns, rainforest preservation or whatever will make a difference and leave our air pure and fit to breathe and the rest of our environment safe and clean.

Finding out more

Friends of the Earth
26-28 Underwood Street
London N1 7JQ
Tel: 081 490 1555

Green Deserts
Rougham
Bury St Edmunds
Suffolk
Tel: 0359 70265

Greenpeace
30-31 Islington Green
London N1 8XE
Tel: 081 351 5100

Further reading

Sara Parkin, *Green Parties - An international guide*, Heretic Books, 1989.

Jonathon Porritt, *Seeing Green*, Blackwell, 1984.

PERSONAL PHILOSOPHY

The development and nurturing of a positive personal philosophy is an important facet of total healthcare. We consciously strive to make our lives fit our own idea of how they should be, and the body is the most immediate physical thing we can mould to fit our desired image.

It is immaterial whether that philosophy is purely in relation to health or more all-embracing; whether it is an individual perspective or shared with a large group. What is important is to have a clear idea of your own purpose and an understanding of how your life works. With this understanding, goal setting, decision making, good health and general life management are all made possible.

Taking responsibility for your own health is an important adult skill. Any philosophy which absolves the individual of this responsibility in my opinion cheats them out of their own growth. Taking responsibility means integrating healthcare into your lifestyle in a beneficial way and taking full possession of your body, the physical reality of who you are.

In the early history of society, health difficulties beyond the individual's own care would be taken to a medicine man or woman, or to the witch doctor. This magic person achieved what healing they could through involving their patient in a truly holistic approach. Special plants, herbs or potions would be given, but a major part of the 'cure' was the dynamic quest or ritual in which the patient would immerse themselves. This meant the psychological and spiritual aspects of the person were wholly focused on cleansing and healing their own body. They were totally involved in their own transformation.

Whilst I am writing this, I am reminded of a recent television programme about giving birth. One of the prospective fathers, on expressing his feelings about the coming birth, said: 'I don't know how it works at the hospital – whether they let fathers stay for the birth, and whether they'll let (my partner) move around in the early stages.' He didn't know whether 'the professionals' would allow this woman to move freely if she felt she wanted to. Who has responsibility here?

Over the last century, particularly during the growth in power of the medical profession, we have all been encouraged to dissociate ourselves from our bodies, to hand over any defective bits to a professional until they can be cured and returned. As a society we desperately need to reclaim our integrity as individuals and recognise our own potential expertise in our own specialist subject – ourselves. Only when we see our bodies as ourselves, as the place where we live, will we be able to claim good all-round health – physical, mental/emotional and spiritual.

Check out your own attitude – what happens when you get a headache or stomach pain? Do you curse the inconvenience and try to remove the problem as you would a stain from a piece of fabric? Or do you stop and ask why this is happening – has your diet been at fault, or your stress level too high, have you been ignoring your body's need for rest? And what do you do? Do you take a pain killer, so that you can stop feeling what is wrong? Or do you seek to resolve what is wrong in the knowledge that if you find and treat the cause of the discomfort then the pain will naturally disappear?

Obviously, allopathic treatments have their place – surgery really is the only life-saving answer for a ruptured appendix (although I must say that the incidence of inflamed and ruptured appendix is significantly lower in those eating wholefood diets), but this way is just another philosophy. We are educated to regard it as the norm, in fact it is one way of looking at healthcare, and to my mind a pretty faulty one. The National Health Service is failing now partly because its premise is incorrect. Suppressing symptoms without recourse to their cause is not health. As a mainstay of our patriarchal society it perpetuates the myth of personal powerlessness. There are strong connections between society as a whole and its institutions. Religious dogmas often seem far removed from the spirituality of their original teachings, and attempts to embrace the individual in social welfare can erode individual rights. Rather than individual freedom, the corner-stone of patriarchy seems to be the removal of personal choice.

Reality is a fact. How we experience it is absolutely up to us – if you imagine reality as a landscape, every philosophy will give you a map or grid to superimpose on the landscape in an effort to make it more understandable. We all use grids or maps, and a conscious knowledge of our own grid (or philosophy) allows us to make sense of our journey.

The more informed we become, the more equipped we are to make choices. In relation to our personal health and welfare, this may mean looking beyond society's main offerings to redefine how our needs may be met. This is an enormous challenge, particularly for those of us who have lived our lives within the security of a narrower outlook. If we believe in the value of our own growth, facing this challenge provides us with a valuable opportunity to take part in our own development; to measure our own nurturing and to participate fully in our own process of transformation.

Further Reading

Neil Freer, *Breaking the Godspell*, Falcon Press, 1987.

Ivan Illich, *Medical Nemesis*, Pelican, 1977.

Anne Wilson Schaef, *When Society Becomes an Addict*, Harper & Row, 1987.

POSTURAL THERAPIES

These are systems of physical realignment in which the emphasis is on re-educating the body's postural muscles.

Alexander Technique works with the conscious holding patterns in muscles to rebalance the whole body with the aim that if the postural muscles are working at their optimum, then ease of movement will naturally follow. The client or student is encouraged to relearn habits of movement through repetition. Holding the body in the 'correct' relaxed position (that which allows the body to move with the most ease), simple movements are repeated until the body learns to do them in an effortless way. This usually involves the presence of the practitioner or teacher exerting some restraining pressure on the body to keep it in the right position.

This form of therapy is popular with actors, musicians and others who use their body as a means of expression, or who do physical work. It originated in Australia where an actor, F.M. Alexander, looked to his body to see what it was he was doing that was causing his difficulties with voice production. Over years of study, he observed the changes in how he held his body – the tense and habitual poses that he struck – and then learned how not to do them.

He observed that healthy children below the age of about three move in a perfectly balanced and co-ordinated way. As they grow older, through imitating their parents, integrating emotions in their bodies, and through faulty experience and poor education, they learn less beneficial body habits. The essence of Alexander technique is in refreshing the body and renewing that childlike ease of movement through conscious control.

One of the first exercises you will learn is how to stand up correctly, without causing strain or discomfort. With the teacher gently holding the head and possibly the back between the shoulder blades, the seated client will stand up and sit down using the leg muscles for power, rather than leading with their head. The teacher ensures that the head is maintained in the midline of the body and that the back is straight. Once learned, the student should be able to feel when they are doing it in the right way.

If you stand up straight and imagine yourself suspended from your sternum or chest bone, you will immediately experience a release of tension in the neck and shoulders. Your chin should be able to settle back a little as your head is then delicately balanced on your neck. This will give you a taste of the physical changes that can occur when your body structure is working at its best.

The importance of a relaxed posture cannot be overstressed. It not only ensures ease of movement, but goes a long way toward preventing some of the structural problems so common in older age. Good posture means there is good tone in the diaphragm, which improves breathing (and voice production) and also assists in abdominal function. Ease of movement means that the body is moving in the way it was designed to, without causing any strain or discomfort or excessive wear and tear on the joints. This all makes it easier to feel relaxed and comfortable in your body.

Treatment from Alexander teachers usually lasts between

thirty minutes and an hour. A full course of these treatments is necessary to learn new postural habits for the whole body and the number involved varies from person to person. When pressed, two Alexander teachers suggested thirty treatments might be an average.

Alexander teachers will often work alongside manipulative therapists like osteopaths and chiropractors, who will be able to correct any structural problems before or early on in a course of treatments. Obviously, postural retraining cannot be successful in the presence of structural misalignment, and there is little point in correcting bony displacements without re-educating the individual so that they need not occur again.

After or during a course of Alexander technique some people feel remarkably changed and physically lighter, while others recognise that they are moving with much greater ease. It is not uncommon, however, to experience aches and pain while the new postures are being learned.

If you have a keen eye, you should be able to spot someone who has done a course of Alexander technique at quite a distance. The way in which they move and a certain quality to their stance marks them out among many others who do not feel so comfortable in their bodies.

Stand up straight and imagine a wire suspended from the heavens and attached to your sternum or chest bone. Feel as the wire is held in good tension how your sternum lifts, taking your whole rib cage along with it. Notice how your whole posture shifts – your weight may settle back into your heels and your arms will feel freer as your whole shoulder and neck area feel less congested. Your neck will also feel as though it is lengthening, and your chin should settle backwards just a little, allowing your head to sit in a more relaxed way upon your neck.

Like Alexander technique, the **Feldenkrais Method** helps retrain the body. An awareness of, and sensitivity to, movement is encouraged through a system of gentle exercises. To take away the pressures of gravity, these are all initially practised with the client or student lying on the ground.

Moshe Feldenkrais used to be an atomic physicist and had studied engineering. A knee injury led him to begin his investigations into the dynamics of movement in the human body. A black belt in judo, he drew on his knowledge of martial arts to develop his method which relates the mechanics of the body to patterns of learning and behaviour. He also worked with F.M. Alexander and explored yoga, psychology and spiritual philosophies. He maintained that in releasing negative physical patterns, restrictive mental patterns would change too.

The method is taught in two ways: awareness through movement is taught in groups, with a teacher leading the class through a range of simple movements. These may be everyday things like flexing the feet, or exercises that are designed to heighten the individual's awareness of the way they use their body. Asked to bend and lower one knee, for example, people may find they tense a number of unrelated body parts like the hands and even the face. Functional integration takes place in individual sessions where the practitioner will interact with and guide the student's body through the range of movements.

These gentle methods can be used by young and old alike, and have been shown to be particularly beneficial for people with special needs. The key to the method is in the conscious awareness of movement and the way this can effect beneficial mental and emotional, as well as physical change.

Finding out more

The Professional Association of Alexander Teachers
Madian
Iorwerth Avenue
Aberystwyth
Dyfed SY23 1EW
Tel: 0970 617586

Society of Teachers of the Alexander Technique
10 London House
266 Fulham Road
London SW10 9EL
Tel: 071 351 0828

The Feldenkrais Method
28A Hampstead High Street
London NW3 1QA

Feldenkrais PTP Information Centre
188 Old Street
London EC1V 9BP
Tel: 081 584 8819

Further reading

F. Matthias Alexander, *The Use of Self*, E.P. Dutton, New York, 1932 (Centreline paperback, 1986).

Moshe Feldenkrais, *Awareness through Movement*, Penguin.

Michael Gelb, *Body Learning: An Introduction to the Alexander Technique*, Aurum Press, 1988.

Glen Park, *Art of Changing*, Ashgrove Press.

Chris Stevens, *Alexander Technique*, Optima, 1987.

Lulie Westfeldt, *F. Matthias Alexander: The Man and His Work*, Centreline Press, Long Beach California, 1984.

QUIET

Mention quiet, particularly to a city-dweller, and a whole host of words spring to mind – peaceful, silence, golden, renewal, relaxation ...

We are exposed to almost constant auditory stimulus, sometimes chosen, sometimes not – like other people's radios, in-store music and traffic noise. When we hear something, it impresses us, makes our mind work to understand, or classify, or make choices about it. I was once appalled to discover, on taking a holiday in a small seaside village, that it took days to clear my head of an assortment of song lyrics, ditties from commercials, hackneyed phrases and background buzz.

Finding a quiet time each day is important, whether we use it to clear our minds, or for more formal reflection or meditation. Without this, our own inner thoughts risk becoming lost in the mêlée of incoming sounds and ideas. Uninvited noise can also be a great irritant, adding to our stress levels and robbing us of the opportunity to relax.

The effects of this type of stress are insidious – we often don't realise how much noise we have tolerated until we quite suddenly notice a silence. Even welcome sounds like music can dull our senses if they become continuous; we can also then become inured to their beauty and less discerning. While we are unconsciously concentrating on blocking out background noises, our bodies can suffer – breathing becomes shallow and there is less available energy for necessary tasks like digestion and repair work.

We all need time alone with our own thoughts and ideas in order to appreciate our own values and validate our beliefs. One wonders at the possibility of original thought while we are constantly bombarded with other people's ideas and society's values, tastes and instructions.

In pregnancy, loud noises and the physical effects of continually resisting low-level noise can cross the placenta. If it troubles the mother, then it can trouble the foetus at a time when it should be allowed to continue its growth uninterrupted.

A quiet time can be one of the most valuable periods of the day, both mentally and physically. Sharing silence with others is a profoundly effective way of improving true communication. We have become very 'sound-reliant'. When we rely on verbal communication it is easy to forget other vital methods of expression. The unspoken communication between lovers and friends is tremendously important and gives us the opportunity to reflect on how we normally convey our thoughts, ideas and feelings. Our body language and the 'vibes' we give off can convey our feelings very well – sometimes very much more clearly than the words we use.

Some of our talk is also necessary only in order to avoid the silence that can make some people feel awkward or vulnerable – we talk and make noise as a protection. It is in silent times that we can heal ourselves; make conscious our inner motivations, and bring creative notions and ideas to fruition. Our selves can be very good company, and if we make friends with ourselves then the quiet time can become rich with the cementing of that relationship.

Some religious houses offer the opportunity of silent retreats; a time to experience this solitary adventure alone or with others. Some may structure the retreats by marking the beginning and the end with some form of ritual, ceremony, or inspirational readings. These can set the tone of the retreat by suggesting a focus, or by unifying the group. The experience of turning inwards in this way, particularly in the company of others, can be remarkably liberating. Those same feelings of uninterrupted communion with ourselves can be experienced in any quiet moments we can find.

Finding out more

National Retreat Association
24 South Audley Street
London W1
Tel: 071 493 3534

The Right To Peace and Quiet Campaign
PO Box 968
London SE2 0RL

Four Winds Centre
High Thicket Rd
Temple Hill
Dockenfield
Farnham
Surrey GU10 4HB
Tel: 025125 4480

Gaia House
Woodland House
Denbury
Nr Newton Abbot
Devon TQ12 6DY
Tel: 0803 813188

RELAXATION

Amidst all the pressures of our hectic lives, we need to find time to relax, but switching off from busy schedules isn't always easy. There is a wide variety of relaxation techniques, from physically based skills which can be utilised in any fifteen-minute gap, to watching hypnotic videos and listening to cassette tapes. The beauty of all skills like these is that once learned, they can easily be used in any available time slots, and once practised the effects are long-lasting.

Relaxation is only possible if we feel safe and secure in our chosen environment. Physical comfort is important – we need to feel free from the restrictions of tight clothing and to be comfortable and warm. Some people, usually those with excess energy, will find it most easy to relax whilst expending that energy physically, so a brisk walk may be the best choice for them. Or that may be a preliminary to any quieter work. Most often, though, full relaxation is a sedentary practice.

When we are stressed, it is more than a feeling of being under pressure – are bodies are affected too. The system will be full of adrenalin, giving that 'all psyched-up' sensation. This is great if we need to meet an immediate crisis, but when sustained for hours, days or months can lead to nervous irritation and physical exhaustion. This can lead us to confuse our bodies further by taking artificial stimulants like caffeine, and this load is compounded by suffering aggravation from an assortment of pollutants. General worries and concerns, unresolved issues and the ups and downs of our emotional responses all add to the stress.

Removing all of these difficulties would be a pretty tall order, but just letting go of our concerns and switching off that ever-ready attitude can be remarkably soothing. It's rather like preparing an elaborate meal – there may be several pots simmering on the stove and a dish in the oven, but it's still necessary to leave the kitchen for a while, even if only to set the table. We may well never get our lives 'just right' or completely stress-free, but perhaps the most useful skill we can cultivate is the ability to switch off from it all and allow ourselves the experience of relaxation and renewal.

Our minds are absolutely capable of juggling a number of projects and we rarely switch off our consciousness altogether. This time off is as essential to our total well-being as any other element of our balanced lives, like periods of leisure and play. Perhaps their most important function is in providing a time for the body and mind to fully unite and heal.

When a muscle is tense it cannot function properly – it can neither receive an adequate blood supply with all the essential nutrients that brings; nor get rid of its waste products. Without these functions, the mechanism of muscle contraction can begin to fail altogether.

A primary concern of most relaxation techniques is to still and quieten the body. This can be achieved in a number of ways, and the simplest is by bringing the areas of tension to our conscious awareness in order that we might then issue the mental instruction to relax. Among the formalised relaxation techniques are **Biofeedback, Autogenic Training** and others which all concentrate primarily on the physical response – it is not easy to relax while a big part of you is tense. There is equipment that can help you recognise tension in the muscles, and a variety of tricks to still the conscious mind. If relaxation therapy is a new idea for you, you may like to begin with the simple techniques described later in this section. There are also relaxation therapists who will be proficient in a number of different techniques to aid relaxation, and relaxation classes are held at many libraries, civic centres and natural health clinics. Here a group of people can go and, sitting in comfort, be talked through the techniques together.

Many people believe in starting at the other end – with meditation or mental focusing exercises – but the aim is always the same; to still and unify the body and mind. If stress is not a chronic problem, there are many everyday pursuits which can aid relaxation including taking holidays, listening to music, becoming engrossed in some creative pursuit or hobby, breathing deeply, walking, dancing, and, of course, simply being quiet.

The comfort of another's touch can be deeply soothing and relaxing, and in this less than tactile world, something we can often miss out on. We often tend to perceive touch as being mainly sexual or familial, but there is a tremendous love to be received and given between friends and partners; simple hugs and physical gestures can make us feel comfortable and easy in ourselves.

Find a comfortable position – either sitting or lying down – and loosen any tight clothing. Make sure you are warm enough and if necessary cover yourself with a rug or similar. Sitting is probably best whilst learning this technique, otherwise there is every possibility of falling asleep. You need to set aside about twenty minutes to do this for the first few times, and once used to the routine will be able to use it in a number of ways: as a five minute pick-me-up; to aid getting off to sleep; or as a full body relaxation taking as much time as you like.

If possible, pick a time when you are not likely to be

interrupted by callers or unwelcome noises, and take the telephone off the hook or switch on the answerphone. For the next twenty minutes or so you are going to concentrate on yourself.

Close your eyes and begin by noticing your breathing – this will begin to focus your attention inside your body. Just become aware of the regular flow of breath into and out of your lungs. Then start to feel the contours of your body as it comes into contact with the chair or the floor and the air around it. Feel your body's weight start to make an imprint as it rests heavily on its supportive surface. This will establish your edges or points of contact with the world and bring your feeling sense into operation.

Now, starting with one foot, squeeze your toes together and let them curl right under themselves. Hold them there for a moment and then relax them. Next, flex your foot, curl your toes in and try to make it as small and tight as possible. Hold for a moment and then relax. Continue on up the leg by squeezing and tightening the calf, knee, thigh and buttock muscles in turn, holding them for a moment and then relaxing them.

At this point you may like to compare the feelings in your legs – the one you have just relaxed may well be feeling heavier, looser and warmer than the other. This comparison is only to reassure your mind that this is a positive and beneficial thing to be doing with your time. You can just enjoy the feelings and carry on the exercise; this time beginning with the toes on your other foot.

Work up your entire body in this way, not forgetting your arms, shoulders (very important!) and your face. This is easy to tense really tight by just exaggerating ugly facial expressions, holding them for a moment, and then relaxing.

By the time you have relaxed your whole body in this

way, you should be feeling quite calm and peaceful inside, and physically loose and relaxed. Take a few minutes to enjoy this and to make sure that you will be able to remember how good it feels. Then open your eyes and remain in your easy, relaxed position for a few minutes before getting up.

You might like to record these instructions on to a tape and play it to remind yourself what to do. As you become experienced at recognising feelings of tension in your body, and more confident in your ability to relax, you may wish to play some tranquil music during your relaxation.

Another simple relaxation technique uses imagery. These focusing exercises can easily transport you to wonderful surroundings where your body and mind can be nourished with beauty and touch, warmed by the sun, or moved by the rhythmic rolling of waves. The mind has amazing power over the body's responses – strongly imaging yourself to be in a place and feeling the emotions and sensations engendered can be as therapeutic as actually being there.

Again, this is something you can think your way through, or script and record. If making a tape, remember to leave time between your suggestions to allow yourself to drink in the surroundings and luxuriate in the feelings. A nice touch is to ask questions, and allow your experience to be different time after time, e.g. you can feel the sunlight on your back as you walk towards the waterfall, what is that you hear? The simplest way to do this is to describe a situation that is peaceful, rich and renewing. It might be totally imaginary, or somewhere you have been or would like to visit.

There are many guided imagery tapes on the market – these are exactly the same thing, only the situation and the cues will then all be given to you.

Further reading

H. Benson, *The Relaxation Response*, Fontana, 1977.

E. Jacobson, *You Must Relax*, Unwin Hyman, 1975.

Louis Proto, *Total Relaxation (The Alpha Plan)*, Penguin, 1989.

José Silva and Philip Miele, *The Silva Mind Control Method*, Granada, 1980.

SKINCARE

The skin is our largest organ of elimination. It plays an important role in continuing good health, yet we take most of its actions for granted. It is our point of contact with the rest of the world, a protective wrapping, the vehicle of our vital sense of touch, and an important temperature regulator. It contains some three million sweat glands, manufactures vitamin D, denotes racial origin and exposure to the sun, and is a mirror of our health.

Weighing some 6–10lbs, and covering about two square yards, this remarkably versatile organ has tremendous powers of elasticity – as witnessed by our ability to grow, put on weight, become pregnant, and even make facial expressions.

We know that our skin is continually renewing itself – losing dead cells and replacing them with new ones. This is part of the process we witness as cuts and wounds heal. The outer layer of our skin, the epidermis, is composed mainly of dead cells, new ones continuously being made in the inner layer or dermis. We naturally shed thousands of these cells each day, but this cycle, like all other body processes, can become sluggish or in need of support. However good our personal hygiene – of course we bathe and clean ourselves – there is always more we can do to encourage healthy skin function.

The skin shares with the lungs the responsibility for

exchanges with the air around us. Your skin breathes too, absorbing oxygen and expelling carbon dioxide formed in the tissues. This explains the great connection between breathing difficulties, like asthma, and skin complaints, like eczema. Looking back through a person's health history, a progression can often be seen from problems in one of these areas to difficulties in another. Long-term smokers often develop dry-skin complaints, and infantile dermatitis, unless properly treated, may disappear only to develop into breathing difficulties as the child grows.

The elimination of uric acid is another skin function (the composition of sweat is virtually identical to urine). The waste we eliminate from the body in perspiration can take some of the pressure off the kidneys and the liver. The more effective ways there are of ridding waste products from the body, the better it can function. Indeed, many healthcare philosophies maintain that insufficient elimination is a major cause of ill health. Getting rid of what is no longer needed in the body is certainly as necessary as providing it with the right nutrients and building materials.

There are enormous benefits to be gained from unclogging the skin by sloughing off the millions of dead cells which can fill the pores. Dry skin brushing is one of the most effective ways I know of doing this, and it has other benefits for the body too – stimulating the lymphatic system and pepping up the circulation. Using a natural bristle skin brush, the whole body is covered with short or long brushing strokes. Starting on the soles of the feet and always working towards the heart, even the scalp can be brushed in this way. Never brush the face, however, as the skin here is too sensitive. The feeling of an all over brush is enlivening and invigorating.

Salts in their many guises form a part of any naturopathic repertoire. Ordinary table salt should not in fact be on any table, but moved to the bathroom, where it is wonderful. A small handful added to bath water is a useful cleansing agent for women, and is particularly helpful if there is any infection or damaged skin. Larger amounts of salt can be used for a salt rub or salt glow. This is tremendously stimulating, sloughing off dead skin cells and giving the circulation a boost:

> Place 2lb of salt in a bowl and add enough hot water to form a thick paste. Taking handfuls at a time, rub well over the whole body for a few minutes – rubbing should be vigorous, but not enough to hurt. Shower off with hot water, and then reduce the temperature to finish off with a tepid or cold shower and gently towel dry. Ideally, follow the salt rub with a short walk or other form of exercise.

This is an excellent cleanser, and can be done once a week as part of maintaining a healthy skin and keeping circulation at an optimum. It can also be used locally on areas of dry skin like feet and elbows: here, though, it is a good idea to follow the salt rub with an application of moisturising oil or cream.

Epsom salts also have a role to play. These are pure magnesium, a mineral required for over 80 per cent of all body activities on a cellular level.

> A hot bath to which 1lb of epsom salts has been added has a wonderfully cleansing effect on the skin, encouraging perspiration and drawing out impurities. As the magnesium is absorbed, it aids the relaxation of muscles, thereby easing any aches and pains. These baths are deeply relaxing and have an important place in any form of stress management.
>
> Ideally, stay in the bath for twenty minutes, and then wrap up warmly and either lie down or go to bed. This ensures that the positive effects of the bath will continue

and the tiredness becomes a benefit – I often recommend these to people who have difficulty relaxing or trouble in getting to sleep.

Epsom salts baths should not be taken if you have eczema, psoriasis or high blood pressure, and women should avoid them during and immediately prior to menstruation as the effects can be depleting at that time. Otherwise, they can be taken up to twice a week.

Simply allowing skin a chance to relax and breathe can be remarkably rejuvenating. A few days off from regularly shaving, or wearing make-up shows instant results in a clearer, healthier looking skin. Air baths are another lovely way of allowing the skin to breathe all over: simply stand near to an open window after a bath or shower, and use your hands to gently massage as much of your body as you can comfortably reach in the stream of (hopefully) fresh air. This gently stimulates all the nerve endings in the skin and results in a glowing feeling all over.

SUPPLEMENTS

In an ideal world, we would be able to obtain all the nourishment we need from the food we eat. Unfortunately, the growing conditions, shipping and storage of fresh food are often geared more towards production targets and ease of transportation rather than to providing and conserving the inherent goodness of the foods themselves.

If you are eating food that is grown more than one mile from the sea, has been stored for more than a few hours or has been treated by freezing, drying or canning, then it will have lost some of its nutrient value. We have farmed the land so intensively in recent years, that many of the nutrients that should be present in the soil have disappeared. Iodine, for instance, is only naturally present in soil from areas next to the sea, otherwise it must be added.

An all-round vitamin and mineral supplement, taken on a regular basis will, as its name suggests, supplement your diet and provide you with essential nutrients. They are not alternatives to a well-balanced diet, but will support those efforts and ensure that a full range of nutritional elements is available to the body. These are the essential building blocks for health. They are necessary for growth, repair and also regulate the metabolism.

The absence of major deficiency of any one can endanger the whole body. The mineral calcium, for example, is necessary for the healthy growth of teeth and bones; vitamin A is essential to the health and structure of the skin and eyes; and vitamin C speeds the healing of wounds through its effects on the cells and blood vessels.

Vitamins and minerals work together in the body: vitamins A and E need each other to work satisfactorily; iron is important in the prevention of anaemia, but it requires an adequate placing of copper to be effective, and this is regulated by the presence of zinc. Iron uptake may be lowered in the presence of tea, coffee and bran, but vitamin C can greatly aid its absorption. This sometimes complicated, synergistic action can be thrown out of balance if one vitamin or mineral is taken in isolation.

While all of us can benefit from a good supply of these materials, certain groups can have greater needs for them, or need them more at particular times in their lives. They are all essential for growing children, but also for women during pregnancy and during the menopause, and particularly if taking the contraceptive pill; for the elderly; for athletes or those making special demands on their bodies; and anybody actively destroying vitamins within their body through smoking, drinking or, in some cases, slimming, or experiencing high levels of stress.

A good multi-vitamin and mineral supplement is the best way to ensure a good supply of all these nutrients. It may provide an excess of some substances, but these are usually easily transported out of the body. Individual vitamins or minerals should not be taken on a long-term basis without professional nutritional advice. They all work together in various ways to ensure optimum health. If one particular nutrient is taken in excess, it can throw the whole system out of balance.

The legacy of poor quality food shows in our overall health, and many health professionals will treat individuals with specific vitamins or minerals in isolation to correct particular imbalances or shortcomings in nutritional status. Those of us without specific health problems that require this sort of treatment will tend to use supplements as an insurance against long-term deficiency, and as a way to maintain optimum health.

You get what you pay for with supplements, and at the cheaper end of the market, additives, synthetic substances and even sugars and saccharine can appear on the list of ingredients. One vitamin C supplement I saw in a high street chain of health food shops contained sugar, orange colouring and orange flavouring alongside a small amount of the vitamin. This makes a nonsense of the whole idea of adding a good, necessary support to your diet.

Some supplement suppliers also use synthetic copies rather than the active vitamins and minerals themselves – these behave differently in the body, and can cause confusion at a biochemical level. If one of the reasons for taking supplements is to increase the body's ability to cope – to relieve stresses – then obviously the natural substance will be preferred.

Most naturopaths and nutritional advisors will have investigated the market and will be able to recommend supplements that are of good quality, additive-free and hypoallergenic (i.e. that the manufacturers will not have used any substances in the packing of the tablets or capsules that are likely to aggravate allergies). They will also suggest, wherever possible, the actual vitamin, rather than a chemical substitute.

Here is a simple table showing some of the actions of vitamins and minerals within the body. It is not a good idea to pick just one or two and take those, without expert advice. If you can identify an area where you suspect you may be experiencing a deficiency, then the best approach is to pick a broad-spectrum supplement which contains a good amount of that substance, or to consult a practitioner. Of course, you could also check that your diet contains adequate amounts of foods that contain it. Vitamins and minerals are usually identified as being present in measurements of milligrams (mg) or micrograms (mcg), although some are measured in international units (IU).

The World Health Organisation has identified minimum daily requirements for many although not all of these micronutrients, and these are known as the Recommended Daily Allowance (RDA). Various studies have shown these figures to be the absolute minimum daily allowance; bearing in mind that we will get some vitamins and minerals from the foods we eat (if we are lucky), I suggest these be used as a minimum figure to look for in multi-supplement tablets.

Care must always be taken during pregnancy, and supplements should not be taken without the advice and monitoring of a healthcare practitioner. There are specific supplement packages on the market for pregnancy, and your naturopath will be able to advise you on these.

Vitamins	Actions	Dietary sources	RDA
A (retinol)	Skin and eyes	Oily fish, green vegetables, yellow fruit, carrots, dairy foods	2500IU
B Complex (B1, B2, B5, B6, B12, biotin, choline, inositol, folic acid, niacin/ nicotinic acid)	All tissue growth, health of skin, mouth eyes and hair, function of nervous system, utilisation of protein, liver function, blood cleanser, aids fertility and	Yeast, wholegrain products, green vegetables, eggs, nuts, some seafood and dairy products, meat	Vary as per vitamin

	digestion of carbohydrates		
C (ascorbic acid)	Health of cells, blood vessels, gums and teeth, wound healing	Raw vegetables, citrus and other fruits, potatoes	30mg
D (chole-calciferol)	Formation of teeth and bones, use of calcium and phosphorous	Sunshine on skin, oily fish, butter, eggs, fish liver oils	100IU
E (tocopherol)	Fertility and muscle health, anti-ageing	Green vegetables, vegetable oils, wheatgerm, nuts	10mg (estimate)

Minerals

Calcium	Function of heart and enzyme re-actions, bones, teeth, blood and nerves	Dairy produce, whole grains, nuts and seeds, green leafy vegetables	500mg
Chromium	Maintains blood sugar levels, helps lower blood cholesterol	Wheatgerm, whole grains, shellfish, brewers' yeast, cheese	200–290 mcg
Copper	Component of many enzymes	Fish, shellfish, vegetables, nuts, whole grains	Less than 1mg
Iodine	Component of thyroid hormones controlling growth and metabolism	Seafoods and seaweeds, produce grown on iodine-rich soils	200mcg

Iron	For haemoglobin to carry oxygen around body, involved in fighting infection	Whole grains, nuts, green vegetables, molasses, dried apricots, meat	Varies through life – needs highest when experiencing blood loss
Magnesium	Growth, repair and maintenance of cells, interacts with calcium	Seafood, nuts, whole grains, dried figs and dates	150–450 mg
Manganese	Growth and development, helps regulate blood sugar, maintains connective tissue	Whole grains, nuts, fruits, avocadoes	2mg
Phosphorus	With calcium for bones and teeth, for release and use of energy	Milk, cheese, eggs, fish, wheatgerm, nuts and meat	1.5–2mg
Potassium	With sodium in regulating body fluids, needed for nerves	Fish, meat, dairy produce, fruits and vegetables, bananas and apricots	2–4mg
Selenium	Resistance to infection and cellular protection	Seafoods, whole grains, cereals, nuts, vegetables, fruits	150mcg
Sodium	Muscle action and balancing body fluids	All vegetables, cheese, salt	2mg

| Zinc | Involved with many hormone actions and in appetite control and hair growth | Offal, shellfish, fish, green vegetables, cereals, meat, pulses | 15mg |

Finding out more

British Naturopathic Association
6 Netherhall Gardens
London NW3 5RR
Tel: 071 435 6464

Green Farm Nutrition Centre
Burwash Common
East Sussex TN19 7LX
Tel: 0435 882482

Incorporated Society of British Naturopaths
Kingston
The Coach House
293 Gilmerton Road
Edinburgh EH16 5UQ
Tel: 031 664 3435

Lambert's Nutritional Suppliers
1 Lambert's Road
Tunbridge Wells TN2 3EQ
Tel: 0892 513116

Nutrition Society
10 Cambridge Court
210 Shepherds Bush Road
London W6 7NJ
Tel: 071 602 0228

Further reading

Dr Stephen Davies and Dr Alan Stewart, *Nutritional Medicine*, Pan Books, 1987.

Earl Mindell, *The Vitamin Bible*, Arlington Books.

Michael Murray and Joseph Pizzorno, *Encyclopedia of Natural Medicine*, Optima, 1989.

Ross Trattler ND DO, *Better Health through Natural Healing*, Thorsons, 1987.

TALKING THERAPIES

Analytic · Cognitive · Behavioural · Humanistic · Gestalt
Transpersonal · Personal Construct · Existential
Process-orientated · Feminist · Transference-based

There are many branches of psychotherapy, all with their own specific techniques, approaches and philosophies. All deal with psychological, emotional and practical difficulties through a variety of talking skills. Sometimes this involves discussing what is happening both in the client's life and in the relationship with the therapist, and having the benefit of the therapist's insights and interpretation. Other times specific skills and techniques may be used to facilitate understanding and change. Common to all these approaches is a desire to help the client manage their lives more effectively, and complete confidentiality.

Throughout our lives we are continually assessing and/or reaching to our effectiveness and our own happiness or contentment. The degree to which we can be successful in our own scheme of things is reliant on a number of different factors. The way we understand the world to be, and our own position in it, colour our actions and expectations as fully as do opportunity and ability. In much the same way as an old injury can be a recurring physical difficulty, so too can an old emotional hurt cause current problems. Psychotherapy can offer a way of reaching back to the cause of any discomfort in a safe supported way and allow healing and understanding.

It is the skills of the therapist and the containment afforded by the commitment to sessions along with the client's willingness to work at taking responsibility for their lives which make psychotherapy so valuable. Many individuals seek out this form of therapy as a powerful aid to personal growth and as a way of effecting and managing change in their lives. In our work to refine the physical, this area of personal experience should not be overlooked both as support and as intrinsic to overall health and well-being.

Most therapists will work with clients on either a short-term contract basis, which is useful for working with specific issues and to allow the establishment of a trusting relationship, or as an ongoing process. An initial commitment is usually required to a mutually agreed number of appointments, although this may be as few as two or three. Some therapists do not charge for the first appointment, because this is really the time when they and the client are interviewing each other and determining whether a commitment to working together would be appropriate.

During this initial meeting, the therapist should be able to explain just how they work, and what you might expect from the sessions. Although psychotherapy can be seen as falling into four main categories: analytic, humanistic, cognitive and behavioural; many therapists use a combination of different approaches in their work. Some work solely with the client's own ideas and experiences, others add their own insights, understanding and interventions.

This is also the time when matters which are important to the client may be raised – their main reasons for entering therapy, specific issues they want to work on, and any relevant experiences they may have of working with others in this way. Any questions about the therapist's training and experience can also be asked. Matters of a more personal nature can sometimes be important when choosing a therapist, and if their political awareness, sexual orientation, or knowledge of a particular area of life would make a difference, then this is the time to enquire about that. Therapists vary in their response to questions such as these, some feeling the client has a right to basic background information; others expressing more of an interest as to why this should be important.

The relationship with one's therapist can be such an important one that it is vital to feel that they can be warm, caring, honest and understanding. This initial interview will be a time when it is necessary to make an initial assessment as to the qualities of the therapist, and whether an ongoing therapeutic relationship would be beneficial.

People often arrive at therapy in crisis and look to receive valuable support, a route to understanding why it has occurred, how to survive it, and a way to make plans for the future. The therapist's role is not to rescue but to help find ways to work with the fabric of an individual's life.

Analytic psychotherapy is based on the findings of Freud and, later, Jung. (See Analysis.) It concentrates on the links between our different levels of awareness and the interplay between our conscious understanding and the workings of the unconscious.

Cognitive psychology maintains that the way we understand the world now is based on the views and assumptions that were generated by previous experiences. By exploring new possibilities and adopting other points of view, we can change our behaviour.

The **Behavioural** approach places more emphasis on the environment. Some of our actions receive rewards, i.e. make us feel good; while other behaviours attract some form of punishment or deprivation. Recognition of these facts and learning more 'good' behaviours can lead to more appropriate ways of acting.

Humanistic psychotherapy seeks to uncover and work with

the unique experience of the individual, affirming their own personal view of the world and strengthening their ability to act from their own truth.

All of these approaches recognise the importance of the mind-body link to varying degrees, and many therapists will place great emphasis on the physical sensations, postures and communications of the client. Although working mainly in the emotional or psychological arenas, psychotherapy recognises the role of feelings in health problems, and that on occasion they may be a cause of physical symptoms.

Depending on the therapist's training, sessions may involve clients enacting old conflicts and finding new resolutions to them; applying a new understanding to established patterns of behaviour, and learning to recognise how habitual responses can colour current attitudes and relationships. Much of this work is uncovered through talking with the therapists, who applies a structure and their own understanding to find some form of resolution. Other techniques may also be used including dream analysis, creative exercises such as movement or painting, and visualisation work. 'Homework' may also be suggested in the form of exercises or pursuits that the client may wish to do to further their progress in between sessions.

Perhaps one of the best-known therapeutic techniques is 'chair' or 'parts' work. This involves inviting an imaginary visitor to the session to sit in a chair near the client. This might be a parent, colleague, friend, or anybody whom the client feels the need to address. Perhaps they need to experiment by telling the visitor something within the security of the session and thereby build up the courage to tell them in real life.

This can be a very useful technique if trying to resolve issues from the past when it would be inappropriate to confront the individual directly, or when it would not be possible to – perhaps because of relocation or death. This can also be a useful way of experiencing and expressing uncomfortable feelings like anger or vulnerability in the safety of the therapy room.

After talking to the 'chair', the client may well be invited to sit there and see if they have any responses to make. This technique can also be used to isolate different aspects of the self, so a facet such as 'critic' or 'ringleader' may be invited to occupy the chair and again some dialogue made possible. This can help to clearly identify different parts of ourselves, and gives the chance to experience a time without the driving force of some aspects of the personality.

Chair work forms a major part of **Gestalt** therapy, which takes place both in individual sessions and in groups. Other forms of therapy may also be extended into a group situation and many therapists run such groups alongside their work with individuals. A common occurrence is for therapists to invite people along to a group after working with them individually for a while. This may mark an end to the individual sessions, or may be an additional support to ongoing work. The group members are usually all working with a particular issue or area of their lives and sharing their experience with others, and hearing their stories can be very beneficial.

Among the many other forms of therapy available are **transpersonal, personal construct, existential, process-orientated, feminist,** and **transference-based**. Transference is an analytic term for the feelings that are projected on to others and, in this case, on to the therapist. Sometimes these can form a strong unconscious bond between individuals, and may be feelings that the client finds too uncomfortable to own for themselves. An awareness of them, and open discussion about them, can be both a liberating and transforming experience.

Many therapists work individually, either in their own homes, or in clinics. Sometimes a group of therapists may band together to form a group practice. Sessions last from between fifty minutes to an hour, and double sessions may sometimes be booked. It is common to have therapy sessions once a week, although twice weekly or more is not unusual, and this can vary between therapists and according to how the process is developing.

A therapist's training involves many hours of individual and group therapy as well as the theoretical content of any course, and most practitioners continue their own personal therapy while they are in practice. They can also receive supervision on their case load from another therapist. Some schools encourage therapists to see clients before they have completed their training, and this work is always carefully supervised by a trainer or lecturer. When working in this way the client will always be informed and a lower fee will be charged.

The rates for psychotherapy vary enormously from practitioner to practitioner. Usually, the more experienced therapists charge more, but a high fee is no guarantee of a better practitioner – there are many other factors to take into account such as their practice costs. Many therapists have a sliding scale of fees, so those on low incomes can still avail themselves of this work.

Finding out more

Association of Group and Individual Psychotherapists
1 Fairbridge Road
London N19 3EW
Tel: 071 272 7013

Association for Humanistic Psychology
26 Huddlestone Road
London E7 0AN
Tel: 081 555 3077

British Association of Psychotherapists
121 Hendon Lane
London N3 3PR
Tel: 081 452 9823

Society for Existential Analysis
Antioch University
Regents College
Inner Circle
Regents Park
London NW1 4NS
Tel: 071 487 7556

United Kingdom Standing Conference for Psychotherapy
167 Sumatra Road
London NW6 1PN
Tel: 071 431 4379

Further Reading

D. Brown and J. Pedder, *Introduction to Psychotherapy*, Routledge & Kegan Paul, 1979.

Irene Claremont de Castillejo, *Knowing Woman*, Perennial, Harper & Row, 1973.

Jay Haley, *Uncommon Therapy*, Norton, 1986.

Strephon Kaplan-Williams, *Transforming Childhood*, Element, 1990.

G. Kelly, *Theory of Personality*, Norton, 1955.

Carl Rogers, *Carl Rogers Reader*, Constable, 1990.

H. Wilmer, *Practical Jung*, Chiron, 1987.

UNDERWATER

Vivation™ · **Aquaerobics** · **Floatation** · **Jacuzzis**

We have looked at hydrotherapy, the use of water internally and externally for its therapeutic benefits. There are, however, many 'immersion' therapies and tools available for pleasure and/or personal growth.

Vivation™ is one such therapy, formerly known as rebirthing. Here, through connected breathing and the support of the practitioner, the client is assisted in releasing negative or pent-up physical and emotional patterns. The ultimate experience is to relive one's own birth and, to this end, sessions will often take place in a specially designed pool, with both practitioner and client in the water. Once the techniques have been learned, and it is possible to let go of today's reality sufficiently to allow earlier feelings to emerge, employing them in water can simulate the warm, watery comfort of being in the womb.

Whether this is actually re-experiencing one's own birth or not, the release of hitherto unexpressed emotions is certainly a form of psychological renewal. Most often, the images which appear to the client during such a session are birth-related – tunnels with a light at the end, being expelled by some unseen force, and entering bright colourful places are common.

Rebirthers or **Vivation**™ practitioners often require some sessions on dry land before progressing to a pool. This is to familiarise the client with the sometimes dynamic nature of the work, and to allow time for the therapeutic relationship to be established. Once learned, the rebirthing techniques and breathing exercises can be practised alone and many people use a morning bath to do this in, feeling that to have begun the day with such a releasing and strong emotional experience prepares them for most eventualities.

This leads to a difficulty I keep hearing about with this type of work. Rebirthers are trained in the techniques and they are indeed dynamic at times. Unfortunately, they often have little or no training in counselling or psychotherapeutic skills. To release feelings that are deep-seated, or that have been around for a long time can be a remarkable experience, but it can also be frightening. It is very important to be able to put such feelings or memories into a safe, productive perspective, and to feel not just relief, but also security after such an episode. I feel the most benefit can be gained from such releases if they are able to be understood and integrated into present reality.

More physically based, the latest beneficial exercise craze is **aquaerobics** – a full-body aerobic working-out in water. The benefits of this are enormous – working the body against the resistance of the water tones muscles much more quickly than any land-based exercise except weight-training. It is gentle on the body, and enables aerobic work and the toning of specific areas without the punishing effects on the joints of conventional high-impact aerobics. And it incorporates all of the fun of messing about in the water.

During a class, the full range of exercises is exhibited by the teacher on the side of the pool and the group in the water follow the teacher's lead. Most of the exercises are performed to music, and because they are performed in the shallow end with the group standing up or holding on to the side of the pool, non-swimmers can join in too. (Non-swimmers should tell the teacher, and may feel more comfortable staying close to the steps for the first few classes.)

The body is so well supported during water work-outs that care must be taken not to overdo the amount of exercise taken initially and also to execute the individual movements carefully as the early signs of muscle tiredness and strain are not so obvious. Information on aquaerobic classes can be obtained from most local authority swimming pools and sports centres.

After each class, there is often time set aside for the participants to swim. This ideal exercise for the whole body makes for a lovely finale to an exercise class and, once again, allows us the wonderful freedom of weightlessness and having fun in the element which supported us throughout our gestation. Spending time in the water is one of the only changes many of us have to relieve the pressures of gravity on our bodies and to experience the freedom that this can engender.

To this end, many people are discovering the benefits of **floatation tanks**. These are rather like large, enclosed baths, filled with warm water and Epsom salts, which allow the body to simply float. Each tank is a light-proof, sound-insulated shell which contains about ten inches of water. The combination of silence, darkness and floating in the warm water generates a deep relaxation, often within minutes of entering the tank. Many people believe that re-experiencing this womb-like situation provides enormous psychological benefits.

Current research shows that the level of relaxation engendered in this environment has deep and lasting effects on stress levels, and can positively influence pain tolerance; this is mainly due to the high levels of natural pain-killers that the body is stimulated to produce. The warm, soothing nature of the experience is extremely comforting, and in allowing the conscious mind to relax, encourages the development of our more intuitive, creative side.

Although most often used for relaxation, floatation tanks provide an ideal situation for creative problem-solving, visualisation work and other forms of self-healing. Extra-ordinary rates of accelerated learning have been noted, using in-tank audio or visual tapes.

The use of floatation tanks can be as regular or intermittent as needed; sometimes more than once a week feels necessary – if working with high levels of stress, for example – whilst at other times a monthly visit can be just enough to keep in touch with the inner calm that is experienced during a float.

Most sessions last an hour, at the end of which the floater is made aware of the time. This is often achieved by music being piped into the tank, before the door is opened. Floaters are not locked in – it is possible to leave at any time, although the most common response is one of surprise that the float is over. People will often say that it feels as though they lost track of time altogether, and that it could have been only a few minutes since they entered the space.

The presence of the salts in the water reduces any risk of infection as well as enabling you to float. Before entering people are requested to shower and to cover any broken skin with plasters or vaseline. The prospect of lying in bath water in which a complete stranger was lying only minutes before, however sanitised the conditions, is not a pleasing one for some people. Aside from the physical situation, there can be the feeling of entering another person's space, or being aware of their energy. To this end, floatation tank managers are usually happy to let you know when the water is changed, and to let you have a copy of their schedule of floats, so a time could be chosen at the beginning of the day or after the tank has had a rest day. Floatation tanks can be found in a variety of health centres and beauty salons, as well as at natural health clinics and specialist float centres.

Another deeply relaxing activity is taking **jacuzzis or spa baths**. They ostensibly work on a more physical level – gently pummelling the body with jets and aerated water – their effects, however, reach far deeper. Some people suggest that the feelings of renewal and healing that can be experienced when bathing in this way are due to subconscious memories of floating in the womb. Others posit that it is because the sea was our ancestral home, and so we are actually reaching back to some distant genetic memory.

The walk-in baths with seating areas around the side seem reminiscent of Roman bathing rituals. Walking into the deep, warm water which can then be brought alive with the press of a button is both stimulating and relaxing. The jets can be aimed at specific body parts for an underwater pressure massage, or one can just float around, being carried in a slow circle by the whirlpool effect. Sitting with warm, swirling water bubbling up to your chin is a delightfully sensual experience.

The continuous action of the water serves as a deep massage, gently stimulating muscles and increasing overall circulation. This effect combines with the heat to have an almost intoxicating effect and care must be taken not to stay in for too long. It is best to get out before you start to feel tired, so that the benefits can continue to be felt rather than just leading you to want to sleep.

In countries with temperate climates, jacuzzis are often sited out of doors, and there are now whirlpool spa adjustments that can be made to regular baths in individual homes, but in the main they are situated at health clubs, gyms and leisure complexes.

Finding out more

British Rebirth Society
18a Great Percy Street
London WC1
Tel: 071 833 0741

Floatation Tank Association
3A Elms Crescent
London SW4

Holistic Rebirthing Institute
23 Albany Terrace
Leamington Spa
Warwickshire
Tel: 0926 882494

VISUALISATIONS

The use of the imagination to create pictures of a desired situation or condition is known as visualisation.

The imagination is one of our most valuable tools or assets, and harnessing its tremendous power can prove to be a truly transformational experience. It is our imagination which allows us to daydream, helps us survive difficult experiences, and can provide innovative solutions to problems. Consciously using it in a structured way provides us with a clear link to our dreams or desires.

There is a technique called Structural Tension, in which that link is invested with the ability to unite our current situation and that which we desire. To use this, you need a clear mental picture of what it is you desire, with as much detail and colour as possible. The technique is a simple one, and its effects can be very dramatic. You establish your current reality – get a clear detailed picture of it – and then see yourself living your dream. Give enough time to each image to allow yourself to really feel what each is like and then move between the two pictures. The to-ing and fro-ing between separate reality sets causes a form of tension which then works to draw the two states closer together.

With any visualisation technique, the more powerful and complete the picture of the desired image, the greater the response. Some people visualise their desires for a few minutes each day, thereby renewing their vision and keeping it as a priority in their lives. You can visualise anything that your imagination will stretch to, and the real purpose of this technique is to centre the attention on a desired goal or change that is actively being worked towards. This can be anything from a career change – when you can picture the new job, work environment, colleagues, what you will be wearing, the journey to and from home – to inner changes in psychological response or emotional patterns.

When beginning to use this powerful technique, it is a good idea to start with something fairly simple, and it is always advisable to pick something that is within one's sphere of influence. Developing the imagination and will is just like developing a muscle; it helps to start in a relatively small way and then build on those early successes.

The body, too, can be affected. Many people work with visualisations to effect changes in shape and immune status. An important part of every exercise in weight training and body building is imaging the effect on the muscle or muscle group that is being worked. Seeing the increase in muscle size and the improved definition of the area in your mind sets up a powerful and immediate connection between mind and body, ensuring that the whole person is focused on the job in hand. Studies have shown that performing the exercises without this mental participation does not result in such good progress.

Our bodies respond fully to our ideas and beliefs of how they should be. When we are happy, we tend to move more freely and easily; without conscious thought. When we smile and laugh a whole range of beneficial physiological changes take place, improving everything from our ability to continue feeling good to our rate of digestion. Visualising ourselves to be in warm, nurturing situations has the same effect as actually being there. This is a common form of visualisation – taking an imaginary journey to a place of beauty and renewal and exploring the beneficial feelings and sensations that engenders. For some this place might be a lush green valley; for others a sun-drenched beach – the focus is on making it as real as possible, wherever it is.

There are lots of relaxation tapes on the market, and many of these include visualisations and guided imagery – these are the same thing, only the ideas and suggestions as to where you are and what sensations you might experience are provided by someone else.

Another beneficial use of visualisations is to imagine the state of our bodies internally. Current research is proving the remarkable effects of visualisation techniques on lowering blood pressure, improving immune status and speeding recovery from illness. Focusing on recovery from a cold, for example, by visualising the mucous membranes slowly drying and the lymphatic system quickly disposing of waste materials, while all your muscles relax, really can make a difference.

When visualisations are used in conjunction with another technique for achieving success, like affirmations, the results can be astounding. One of the best ways I know of combining these two powerful aids is to spend some time visualising my desire each day (a completed book, for example) and then devising an affirmation to support this, perhaps: 'Today's the day I complete the book.' Repeating the affirmation at times throughout the day continues the work of the earlier imagining. I also repeat the visualisation at the end of the day.

If you want something to happen, it makes every sense to concentrate and use every possible aid to achieve it, and unlocking the powers of imagination yields tremendous benefits as it overflows into other areas of your life and re-establishes the connections between what you think, who you are and what you do.

Further reading

Richard Nelson Bolles, *What Colour is your Parachute*, Ballantine Books, New York, 1979

Kenneth Meadows, *The Medicine Way*, Element Books, 1990.

Barbara Sher with Annie Gottlieb, *Wishcraft*, Ballantine Books, New York, 1979.

WOMEN

Women's healthcare is an area where natural therapies and techniques can be particularly beneficial. There are some good hydrotherapy measures for enhancing vaginal health, and the acidity of the body, which is determined to a large part by diet, can directly influence the incidence of disturbance in this area. (The pH or acidity of the vagina is inversely proportional to the pH of the rest of the body – when the body is slightly alkaline, as it should be, the vagina becomes slightly acidic. This makes it an unwelcome place for thrush and other invading organisms.)

The problems of painful, absent or heavy periods respond well to herbal and naturopathic treatments; their gentle effects encouraging the body to find its own natural balance. Menstruation has a negative image for some people, and the combination of positive supportive measures and counselling can reinforce the beneficial potential of this special time. The monthly cycle also provides a good sense of timing on which detoxification programmes and health regimes can be based.

Menopause is another major event in a woman's life when natural healthcare methods can be both useful and effective. Simple measures such as establishing a regular habit of weight-bearing exercise prior to menopause can greatly reduce the risks from osteoporosis (thinning of the bones). There are many dietary measures, herbs and supplements that can also assist with the transition and aid the body to rebalance itself. Counselling or therapy specifically geared towards exploring the changes in internal and external status can be particularly helpful.

Natural contraception and fertility control are among a range of self-care approaches. This method of pin-pointing the fertile time in each cycle can help relieve couples of the burden of full-time contraception, or, indeed, aid them in their attempts to conceive. Every month, at the time of ovulation (i.e. when the woman becomes fertile) there are changes in both her basal or resting temperature and the mucus secretions of her vagina. These can both be measured quite easily. The basal temperature can be taken immediately on waking each morning, and the vaginal secretions tested for viscosity or stickiness. Noted over a couple of months, it is soon easy to see what point ovulation occurs, even for those with irregular cycles.

The only difficulty with this method is that sex can interfere with it! The presence of secretions and creams, etc. in the vagina can upset the mucus reading, and the excitement of a relationship can alter the basal temperature. If this is the case, the findings may need to be charted over a longer period of time for a clear pattern to emerge. Nowadays, this natural method may be less than useful as a means of contraception because of the need for protection from disease which only the barrier methods and safer sex practices can provide.

A number of women record the changes in their cycle even though they are not sexually active. Should a relationship develop, they even have a strong record to refer to, but perhaps more important is the feeling of knowing one's own body a little better.

Regular breast checks and even gynaecological self-examination are further examples of this wise concern over how our bodies function. It is a good idea for women to examine their breasts each month, ideally just after a period or on a fixed date so that any changes in breast appearance and texture can be detected. It can also help in reuniting us with this part of our bodies.

Unless breast-feeding or in a sexual relationship, it is very easy not to pay any attention at all to our 'sexual' areas and I feel this diminishes us. In 1990, the UK Government advised women that self-examination was a waste of time. This really has to be one of the most irresponsible statements I have ever heard, and I am glad to say that many women are choosing to disregard it. The statement was issued at a time when there were over 150,000 women with breast cancer in Britain, and this country has the highest mortality rate for this type of cancer in the world. Early detection saves lives – alerts us to the problem before it becomes too entrenched, too difficult to resolve. If you find a lump or something unusual in your breast it is not likely to be serious, but if it is then early treatment is the best course of action.

Well-illustrated leaflets on breast examination can be found at most health clinics and well-woman centres. Speculums for gynaecological self-examination can be bought at any chemist, and again many clinics can advise on their use for those who have never been examined with one. A mirror and some photos of healthy vaginas and cervixes are all that is needed. This is not a substitute for regular pap or smear tests, rather as good an idea as routinely cleaning behind one's ears.

Natural childbirth is a rapidly growing choice for women in the West. Deciding to allow the body's own pain-killers to do their work is an obvious choice for a healthy woman – pharmaceuticals and surgical intervention have their place in emergencies. I am not advocating painful delivery, but more and more women are discovering that if they are relaxed, and have support during labour and have prepared themselves by learning breathing and focusing techniques, then such interventions may not be needed.

There are many birthing classes around the country which

include prenatal exercises to help stretch the ligaments and improve muscle tone. It is often easier to get back into shape after delivery if you remain active during pregnancy, and these exercises can also help make the birth easier.

Another important factor is the choice of location –some women feel more relaxed by the prospect of a home delivery, while others prefer the reassurance of a hospital birth. Although it is important to consider the potential risks as well as the benefits when deciding where to have a baby, women should always have the choice – in many areas the medical profession tries to make it difficult for women who choose a home delivery. Not only, then, must the decision be made as early as possible, but it may also be necessary to employ an independent midwife if a home birth is wanted.

The National Childbirth Trust is a wonderful resource for more detailed information, and their counsellors can also help with any breast-feeding queries and information on baby allergies (one of the most common allergies in babies is to cows' milk!).

There are a number of herbs which can be taken as teas during the later stages of pregnancy to help delivery. Individual assessment is necessary to ensure their safety and efficacy, but both raspberry leaf and lady's mantle can be taken once a day when the birth day is due. A cup of either tea, slipped slowly while it is still warm, can help relax the abdominal muscles and reduce tension.

Many women find that hydrotherapy can also be useful both during and after the birth – warm, moist towels placed over the diaphragm in the early stages of labour can help relieve the pain of contractions; and massage of the abdomen, shoulders and low back can be a comfort. It is well worth consulting a naturopath or a well-woman centre if a home birth is desired.

Breast Examination

Set aside fifteen to twenty minutes for the first few monthly examinations, after that they can be completed in about five minutes. The best time is a few days after menstruation, or, if you do not have periods, then on a regular date each month. Initially, this will be a process of familiarising yourself with the general appearance of your breasts, any unusual puckering or changes in fullness will then be more easily apparent.

Begin by looking at your breasts when standing in front of a mirror. Note their asymmetry, their contour, the positioning of your nipples and their overall appearance. Look at both side views and then lean forwards towards the mirror and again observe the general outline of your breasts as they fall away from your chest wall.

Next, lie down on your back and bend one arm, placing the hand underneath your head. This allows full access to the breast and armpit for your other hand. Using the flat of your fingers held together, make small circular pressing movements on the outermost border of your breast. Work your way around the outside of your breast, and include an investigation of your armpit, until a full circle is completed. Continue covering your breast in this way, making smaller and smaller circles until you reach your nipple.

Notice the colour and appearance of your nipple and its hardness, then repeat the procedure on your other breast.

Most breasts feel glandular or bumpy when examined in this way, and with practice you will soon be able to differentiate between what is normal for you and any changes in texture or feel.

Finding out more

Active Birth Centre
55 Dartmouth Park Road
London NW5
Tel: 071 267 3006

Association for Improvements in the Maternity Services
163 Liverpool Road
London N1 ORF
Tel: 071 278 5628

Breast Care and Mastectomy Association
26a Harrison Street
London WC1H 8JG
Tel: 071 837 0908

National Childbirth Trust
Alexandra House
Oldham Terrace
London W3 6NH
Tel: 071 992 8637

Terrence Higgins Trust
52–54 Gray's Inn Road
London WC1X 8SO
Tel: 071 242 1010

Women's Health Information Centre
52 Featherstone Street
London EC1Y 8RT
Tel: 071 251 6580

Women's Training Assoc.
5 Spennithorne Road
Skellow
Doncaster DN6 8PF
Tel: 0302 337151

Further reading

Janet Balaskas and Yehudi Gordon, *Encyclopaedia of Pregnancy and Birth*, Little, Brown 1992

Janet Balaskas, *New Active Birth*, Harper Collins 1992.

The Body Shop, *Mamatoto, A Celebration of Birth*, Virago, 1991.

Irene Claremont de Castillejo, *Knowing Woman*, Harper & Row, 1973.

Federation of Womens Health Centres, *How To Stay Out of the Gynaecologist's Office*, Woman to Woman Publications.

Dr Michelle Harrison, *Self Help With PMS*, Optima, 1991.

Angela Phillips and Jill Rakusen, *Our Bodies, Ourselves*, Penguin, 1989.

Penelope Shuttle and Peter Redgrove, *The Wise Wound*, Paladin 1986.

(e)XERCISE

Exercise works the most important muscle in the body – the heart. As we work individual muscles or muscle groups, we improve the heart's capacity and ability to pump. This improved blood supply enables the muscles to work well and grow, and the general circulation is improved too. Although blood is pumped around the body, the lymphatic system (a fundamental part of our immune response and necessary for the removal of toxins) depends upon the mechanical effects of movement.

In order to strengthen the heart muscle, improve lung function, pep-up the circulation and the lymphatic system in this way, twenty minutes' exercise three times a week is necessary. To begin with, five minutes every day, or six days out of seven, is a good introduction and will establish some form of exercise as a regular part of your daily routine. This also begins to stretch your body's capacity for exercise, preparing you for increased work as your fitness improves. This ability increases very quickly. The effects of sustained and regular exercises are amazing: within days it becomes clear to see how stamina, strength and suppleness are increasing. It's almost as if these muscles have all been ready and waiting to be stretched and tested, their response is so rapid.

For some, exercise is seen as a chore, and the only way to transform this into the life-enhancing event it should be is to find an enjoyable, interesting way to work-out. The options are legion.

If you enjoy nature, brisk walks may be the perfect way to begin any fitness campaign. Walking is an excellent all-round exercise that can improve muscle tone throughout the body; even peristalsis (the way food is moved through the gut) can be improved by regular walks. The abdominal muscles are gently squeezed and stretched with every step, and walking uphill is the most effective for toning this area. This also makes the leg muscles work even harder. Wherever possible, walking on grass gives the best results because it gives a little when you put your weight down (sand has a similar quality).

Walking, and indeed all weight-bearing exercises, can be an important aid to women. Osteoporosis is a condition that can affect post-menopausal women – it causes the bones to become thinner and more brittle, so they fracture more easily. Regular weight-bearing exercise before, during and after the menopause has been shown to reduce the risk of suffering in this way.

Many people find that it is the social content of any activity that they enjoy the most. There are many contact sports that absolute beginners can join in with – they aren't all designed for professionals. Most small towns, community centres and even some firms have their own football, netball, rugby or rounders teams. Joining a sports and social club is a good idea in smaller communities and most gyms will at least have a snack or juice bar where people can meet. The advantages of joining a centre like this range from club tournaments, which pit whichever members choose to sign on against each other, to the spontaneous situations which often arise when someone needs a partner for tennis or an opponent for squash.

If time is an important consideration, there are many exercises that can be done at home. An exercise bike in front of an open window, or a bouncer (mini-trampoline) can provide a good aerobic work-out at any point during the day. There is a range of exercise videos available that cover a wide variety of approaches – from Callanetics to cardiac funk.

If you like dancing, then there are always discos and clubs to go to, or for a more social element there is a range of classes from jive and jazz to traditional Irish dancing. Exercise doesn't have to be all about sweaty bodies in bare-walled gymnasia; and you don't have to hurt to get fit.

If you would prefer a solitary pursuit, however, weight training is *all* about sweaty bodies in gyms. This form of work-out is one of the most richly and immediately rewarding exercises I know of – after only a few weeks of body building you can see obvious visible changes in the size and shape of your whole body. After only a few sessions you can start to feel the difference. Initially this requires a strong commitment to visiting a gym four times a week for work-outs, but very soon it can become positively addictive. The natural pain-killers (endorphins) produced by the body, along with their mood-changing effects and the fact that appetite is suppressed for a few hours after each work-out, result in incredible 'highs'. The same feelings are experienced by long-distance runners, joggers and all athletes who work their bodies continuously. These feelings must contribute to the easy, swinging gait, bounce in the step and proud posture of all those who exercise regularly.

Whatever form of exercise you choose, it is important to ensure that you are properly equipped. This doesn't only apply to specialist pursuits like rock climbing or scuba diving – walkers need proper shoes; cyclists really need safety helmets and, if cycling through traffic, face masks to limit the amount of poisons they inhale. Weight-trainers and others using any type of machinery or gym equipment must be properly trained in their use to ensure good results as well as safety.

Those choosing activities that include any form of jumping – from high-impact aerobics to jogging, need to ensure the safety of the surface and the protection of their shoes. Well-sprung floors in dance studios and gyms do much to cushion the joints, but proper footwear is essential. Jogging on grass is much safer and a better exercise than running on concrete or stone. Every sport or exercise has its own guidelines and necessities, and finding out about these before you start can guard against many injuries.

All exercising requires a warm-up period, or some sort of preparatory movement. Usually these are gentle stretching and toning exercises and they can form an enjoyable routine in their own right, especially if done to music or in the company of others. They can also be a good way to zero in on any specific body areas that need extra attention – the abdominal muscles, for example – and are excellent for improving suppleness generally.

Movement is a true sign of life. Positively one of the best ways to maintain our 'aliveness' is through exercise. It maintains the mobility of our joints, helps regulate the metabolism, improves muscle tone and size, increases our oxygen capacity and improves posture. Exercise lets our bodies work more efficiently – we feel better and look good.

Finding out more

The Sports Council
16 Upper Woburn Place
London
Tel: 071 388 1277
Regional branches in local telephone directory.

YAWNING/GROANING

Yawning is the body's way of getting more oxygen. It is usually a sign that we are tired and need the additional energy that a deep intake of air will provide, or that for some other reason the body has not been receiving enough oxygen and needs more. Smokers yawn more than non-smokers, and when we are tense we need those additional deep breaths because the body is working hard against the structural resistance of tight muscles.

A good yawn also means a longer than usual exhalation, thus ridding the body of used or de-oxygenated air at a much faster rate than usual. One of the most immediate physical effects of stress is that our breathing becomes shallow; we may often be surprised to find ourselves yawning whilst concentrating hard on a particular job or task. Taking regular breaks from any activity, particularly if sedentary, enables us to regulate our breathing again. A simple stretch will open up the ribcage, and just walking around for a moment or two will return things to normal.

Groaning is a wonderful technique for increasing oxygen intake and destressing the entire body. This simple easy activity releases any pent-up emotional energy as well as getting rid of any tensions. It is particularly useful at the end of a hard day or after any period of intense concentration.

It is best to lie on the floor to do this, although if floor space is limited, a bed or tabletop will do just as well. Take a deep breath in and, instead of breathing out as you would normally, groan it out. (A company director I taught this to was once discovered by bemused colleagues lying on the boardroom table!)

At first it feels and sounds rather strange and you need to stick with it for a few breaths before the self-consciousness disappears, and then it seems to come naturally. You will find yourself groaning away any frustrations, muscle tensions and bad feelings. The tone and loudness of the groaning will modulate, and you may find some groans lasting longer than others. It becomes easy to lose track of time and just give yourself up to the feeling. Groaning has its own natural cycle and you will quickly reach a point where you have nothing left to groan away!

Beyond getting rid of unwanted stresses, this is also a very enpowering technique which should leave you feeling envigorated and refreshed.

ZYGOMA

This is a cheat of an entry to allow me not only to complete the promise of the title, but also to include one of my favourite natural therapies.

The zygoma or zygomatic arch is commonly known as the cheek bone. Its covering of muscles and facial skin is fully exercised in the supremely pleasurable activity of laughing. Laughter is wonderful therapy – in every sense of the word. You can do it anywhere and at any time. It exercises your body beautifully, promotes the release of mood-enhancing chemicals in your brain and, depending on your timing, can infuse others with the same sense of joy and mirth.

As well as being fun, laughing exercises the neck, the muscles of the chest wall and the diaphragm, and ensures that the stomach and the liver, spleen and other organs are gently massaged. With the diaphragm acting as a pump, fresh nutrients and oxygen supplies are speeded around the body and peristalsis (the way food naturally moves through the gut) is improved. Genuine laughter also increases the level of an antibody in the saliva – IGA – which helps protect against colds and flu.

There is a meditation technique based on laughing which builds on its infectious quality and as such is often most effective when used in groups, at least initially. It serves as an introduction to feeling really in touch with our true feelings and provides a good contact with the energy centre in the abdomen.

Participants start laughing, usually in response to the teacher's own laugh, and soon find it very easy to keep going, prompted by the laughter around them. At a given point they stop and immediately close their eyes and focus their attention on the centre of their bodies. The release of emotion through laughter makes for easy access to the stillness which is to be found within all of us. People's responses are of recognising that calm and contacting feelings of joy, stillness and peace within themselves.

For centuries we have known about the importance of our state of mind and its connection with good health. An optimistic attitude truly is a life-saver, and finding humour in a situation can provide a myriad of immediate benefits too.

A simple smile can positively affect your health. The facial muscles exert a direct influence on an area in the brain called the limbic system. This group of glands acts as a switchboard, regulating the speed that nerve impulses are transmitted and thereby controlling the level of performance of both mind and body. All the nerve messages from throughout the body must pass through this system and smiling has the effect of speeding their passage by increasing the number of neurotransmitters, the chemicals which carry the messages.

AND FINALLY...

This book contains a reservoir of health-giving alternatives for those with any specific complaint, which can also be dipped into for a wealth of ideas on lifestyle change and the promotion of full health.

Prevention is the key to continued good health. Prevention from disease can be affected by specific measures; prevention of the states that predispose an individual to disease is the real scope of naturopathy – stepping in before problems appear. If we support our bodies and the way they naturally function, then many of our so-called civilised disorders begin to recede. The degenerative diseases so common in middle and later ages are in part directly attributable to our lifestyle in earlier years.

An important aspect of naturopathy is its role in ongoing health education. Although most people arrive at a naturopath's office with specific disorders, a growing number of individuals are arranging consultations while in good health; wanting advice on improving their constitution, ensuring continuing optimum health, or on how to encourage full health in their children. This points to a new way for individuals to take power and control in their own lives and manage their own health and well-being.

I can think of few things more stressful than trying to follow all of the suggestions in this book at once or to experience all of the therapies. If something seems like good, common sense then try it out. The information and resources given should be enough to guide you, and I hope you will find that most of the measures contained here are rooted in good common sense. They also embrace fully the holistic synthesis of mind, body and spirit, working together to affirm their unity and the integrity of individual experience.

Through information we gain the freedom to make choices, and informed choice is fundamental to sovereignty over our own bodies, our own lives. Reflexologists may access the unified organism through the feet, aromatherapists via the nose – in many cases the choice rests with you.

OTHER USEFUL ADDRESSES

Appropriate Health Resources and Technologies Action Group
1 London Bridge Street
London SE1 9PG
Tel: 071 378 1403

Balcombe Books
PO Box 101
Epsom
Surrey KT19 9UY

Bartragh Centre
Bartragh Island
Lillala Bay
County Mayo
Eire
Tel: 010 353 96 32285/32514

The Bates Association (eyesight care)
Friars Court
11 Tarmount Lane
Shoreham-by-Sea
West Sussex BN43 6RQ

The Breakthrough Centre
7 Poplar Mews
Uxbridge Road
London W12 7JS
Tel: 081 749 8525

Confederation of Healing Organizations
Brundenell House
Quaniton
Aylesbury
Bucks
Tel: 029675 250

Cortijo Romero (holidays)
72 Meadowsweet Road
Creekmoor
Poole
Dorset BH17 7XT
Tel: 0202 699581

Council for Complementary and Alternative Medicine
179 Gloucester Place
London NW1 6DX
Tel: 071 724 9103

Findhorn Foundation
The Park
Forres
Scotland IV36 0TZ
Tel: 0309 73655

Institute for Complementary Medicine
Unit 4
Tavern Quay
Rope Street
Rotherhithe
London SE16
Tel: 071 636 9543

Society of Students of Holistic Health
160 Upper Fant Rd
Maidstone
Kent ME16 8DJ
Tel: 0622 29231

Tigh na bruaich
Shruy by Beauly
Inverness-shire IV4 7JU
Tel: 0463 76254

Tyringham Naturopathic Centre
Newport Pagnell
Buckinghamshire MK16 9ER
Tel: 0908 610450

More titles in the Alternative Health series

Aromatherapy by Gill Martin

Aromatherapy uses the essential oils of plants, which are massaged into the skin, added to baths or taken internally to treat a variety of ailments and enhance general well-being.

Price £5.99

Encyclopaedia of Natural Medicine by Michael Murray and Joseph Pizzorno

The Encyclopaedia of Natural Medicine is the most comprehensive guide and reference to the use of natural measures in the maintenance of good health and the prevention and treatment of disease. It explains the principles of natural medicine and outlines their application through the safe and effective use of herbs, vitamins, minerals, diet and nutritional supplements, and covers an extensive range of health conditions, from asthma to depression, from psoriasis to candidiasis, from diabetes to the common cold.

Price £13.99

Chiropractic by Susan Moore

This guide to chiropractic concentrates on the actual treatment itself, seen from a patient's point of view. In a straightforward way, it answers all your questions about chiropractic, as well as providing background information about this popular therapy.

The author is a practising chiropractor, well aware of the concerns of first-time patients.

Price £5.99

Herbal Medicine by Anne McIntyre

Herbal medicine has been known for thousands of years. It is an entirely natural system of medicine which relies on the therapeutic quality of plants to enhance the body's recuperative powers, and so bring health – without any undesirable side effects.

Price £5.99

Alexander Technique by Chris Stevens

Alexander Technique is a way of becoming more aware of balance, posture and movement in everyday activities. It can not only cure various complaints related to posture, such as backache, but teaches people to use their body more effectively and reduces stress.

Price £5.99

Massage Therapy by Adam Jackson

A natural, safe and extremely effective therapy for everyone, it can be used as an aid to training in sport, in promoting healing after injury or as a relaxation technique. Massage therapists work with footballers, weightlifters, athletes, alongside chiropractors and osteopaths, in hospitals or even assisting with the tensions in the boardroom.

Iridology by Adam Jackson

Iridology is an ancient diagnostic technique through analysis of the iris of the eye. It is painless, non-invasive, and an astonishingly accurate method of health analysis which reveals the condition of each and every organ in the body. Iridologist Adam Jackson explains in a straightforward way how iridology works, what the basic markings and colours in the iris mean, and provides a guide to self-analysis.

He also outlines how to design a personal preventive healthcare programme using diet, exercise, stress management and natural therapies.

Price £5.99

Healing the Heart by Elizabeth Wilde McCormick

Every year in Britain 175,000 people survive heart attacks. But heart disease accounts for one in three deaths in the Western world and is the biggest killer in our society.

Drawing on recent, ongoing research into the effects of stress on the body, and the heart in particular, this book balances clinical fact with psychological considerations, linking mind, body and spirit. Taking a holistic approach, it explores how stress and unhappiness can harm the heart, and how underlying psychological issues have to be tackled along with the physical care of the heart.

Price £5.99

Shiatsu by Ray Ridolfi

This is a fascinating guide to the ancient art of Shiatsu.

Ray Ridolfi is a practising Shiatsu therapist and is well aware of the particular concerns of first-time patients. He has written a guide full of practical and straightforward advice as well as providing background information about this increasingly popular treatment.

Price £5.99

Healing Hands by Allegra Taylor

In this book, Allegra Taylor explores the potential we all possess to develop and channel our healing energies for the benefit of ourselves and our friends and family. Drawing on her experience as a practising healer, she dispels the myths surrounding healing and explains in a down to earth way the nature of the healing energy that surrounds us.

Many techniques – from crystals to visualization to aromatherapy – are detailed, along with practical guidelines to good health and wholeness.

Price £5.99

The Bates Method by Peter Mansfield

The Bates Method is a non-invasive and natural way of enhancing perception and relearning how to see, using simple and enjoyable techniques to relieve strain and improve brain/eye co-ordination.

Peter Mansfield, a practising Bates Method and Alexander Technique teacher, draws on a wide range of the therapeutic and educational experience in his introduction to this fascinating holistic approach to good sight.

Price £5.99

All Optima books are available at your bookshop or newsagent, or can be ordered from the following address:

Little, Brown and Company (UK) Limited,
PO Box 11
Falmouth
Cornwall TR10 9EN

Alternatively you may fax your order to the above address.
Fax number: 0326 376423

Payments can be made as follows: cheque, postal order (payable to Little, Brown and Company) or by credit cards, Visa/Access. Do not send cash or currency. UK customers and B.F.P.O. please allow £1.00 for postage and packing for the first book, plus 50p for the second book, plus 30p for each additional book up to a maximum charge of £3.00 (7 books plus).

Overseas customers including Ireland, please allow £2.00 for the first book plus £1.00 for the second book, plus 50p for each additional book.

NAME (Block letters) ....

ADDRESS ....

....

I enclose my remittance for _____

I wish to pay by Access/Visa Card

Number | | | | | | | | | | | | | | | | |

Card expiry date